Leon Chaitow is a registered osteopath and naturopath, editor of the *Journal of Bodywork and Movement Therapies*, and Honorary Fellow and former senior lecturer at the University of Westminster, London. Author of more than 60 books, including *Holistic Pain Relief*, he lectures internationally on both bodywork and general health topics from an integrated perspective.

LEON CHAITOW

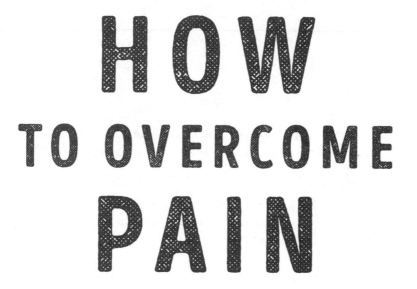

HOW
TO OVERCOME
PAIN

Natural approaches to dealing with
everything from arthritis, anxiety and
back pain to headaches, PMS and IBS

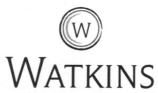

WATKINS

Sharing Wisdom Since
1893

This edition first published in the UK and USA in 2017 by
Watkins, an imprint of Watkins Media Limited
19 Cecil Court
London WC2N 4EZ

enquiries@watkinspublishing.com

1 3 5 7 9 10 8 6 4 2

Designed and typeset by Clare Thorpe

Printed and bound in Finland

A CIP record for this book is available from the British Library

ISBN: 978-1-78678-017-1

www.watkinspublishing.com

This book is dedicated to my wife Alkmini
with love and thanks

CONTENTS

INTRODUCTION

Pain is an inevitable and universal experience – it affects us all at some time. Of course, the pain we most often experience is acute but transient and short-lived – a self-limiting event. A cut, a bruise, a sting, even a break – all are dealt with by our body's self-repair mechanisms.

Chronic pain takes pain into another dimension altogether – and can be experienced as a crushing life sentence. We need to be reminded that the body's self-regulation (technically known as homeostasis) also operates constantly in chronic settings, just as it does in acute ones. Indeed, some of the body's repair mechanisms – such as inflammation – are themselves a source of pain, even though they are helping to heal. This highlights a point that this book tries to emphasize: the more you understand about the causes and mechanisms that produce pain, the more you will be able to modify or eliminate it.

Chronic pain can be seen as a burden or a challenge. How you manage your pain is, to a very large extent, up to you. Another of the primary objectives of this book is to show you ways to approach your pain positively, enabling you to lead as normal a life as possible. A key message to that end is "Hurt does not necessarily mean harm." In other words, even though it hurts, try to carry on as normal (walking, working, gardening and so on), unless you have been specifically advised to avoid particular activities. Using our pain as an excuse to retreat from performing everyday tasks leads to a spiral of inactivity, increased disability and loss of self-confidence.

An important first step in reversing such a tendency is to learn as much as possible about your pain. If you understand why you are feeling pain, and are aware of the possibility of recovery, you will manage the situation far more positively than if you do not understand the processes and suffer from feelings of anxiety and helplessness that amplify the pain.

Having worked as an osteopathic practitioner in private, as well as state-funded, practices in the United Kingdom, and also in southeast Europe, I have been fascinated to observe the differences in patients' coping skills, both within and between these settings. Much of my work has been with people who are in considerable and often permanent pain, suffering from conditions such as arthritis and fibromyalgia. One clear impression I have gained, supported by medical research, is that learning about his or her own condition often helps the person in pain as much as any treatment. Knowledge is power, and understanding your pain gives you power over it.

One of my motivations in writing this book was to bring to a wider audience as much information as possible about pain, based on current research (as well as effective traditional methods), and to show what we can do to help ourselves to recover from pain, or to cope with it. The sheer range of causes, types and intensities of pain, and of ways in which it can be modified, blocked, eased or eliminated, is beyond the scope of any one book. What can be done here is to convey the essence of the pain story, giving you the knowledge that will empower you to deal with your inevitable periods of pain most appropriately. Instead of "no pain, no gain", this book aims to give you "more information, less pain".

LEON CHAITOW D.O.
www.leonchaitow.com

UNDERSTANDING YOUR PAIN

Of all symptoms, pain is the one that is most likely to drive you to consult your doctor. Acute pain is a warning that alerts the defence and self-regulating mechanisms of the body that the brain senses danger. Without acute pain you would not remove your hand from a flame. When a fire alarm rings, finding the source of the fire is far more urgent than switching off the alarm. But when pain is chronic, as it often is, the causes are seldom obvious.

Understanding how chronic pain evolves, and how it may be modified, are the major aims of this book. We now know that "pain is in the brain", and should remember that what we "feel" depends on how the brain interprets and gives meaning to the multiple messages it receives. We can learn from most chronic pain; and we may be able to ignore it safely, manage or successfully treat it in a variety of ways. This book will explore all these options.

WHAT IS PAIN?

Initially, pain serves as a message of distress, danger or damage – a call to protect the area that hurts that is interpreted in the brain as "pain".

Something will have happened to stimulate or irritate tiny nerve structures called nociceptors (pain receptors) – possibly inflammation, chemical irritation, heat, or a mechanical event, such as pressure, stretching, cutting or tearing. The resulting pain messages travel to the brain via mylenated (sheathed) nerves, which carry impulses rapidly at 65½ft (20m) a second, and unmyelenated nerves, which carry impulses at 6½ft (2m) a second.

Nociceptors are found in most tissues of the body, in greater numbers where we are most sensitive. Each nociceptor has a threshold

HOW WE FEEL PAIN
Pain messages travel from the site of injury to the brain, where pain is experienced through a virtual body map.

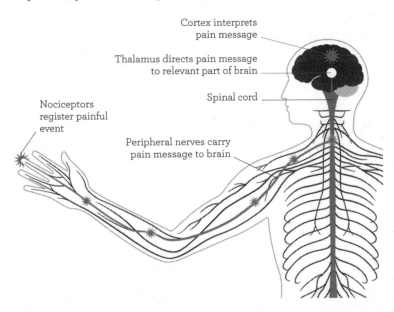

Cortex interprets
pain message

Thalamus directs pain message
to relevant part of brain

Spinal cord

Nociceptors
register painful
event

Peripheral nerves carry
pain message to brain

that has to be exceeded before it reports to the brain that there is a problem. This threshold varies widely, with a number of factors contributing to what the individual "feels", and how he or she interprets that feeling. A major reason for the pain threshold changing is a process known as sensitization, which is explained later in the book (see pages 21–4).

Although the alarm messages that we perceive as pain usually start in the part that hurts, this is not where we actually feel pain. Instead, pain is felt in the brain, by means of a virtual body map (the homunculus) that resides there. If this seems strange, consider that many amputees feel "phantom"pain in the missing limb, long after it has been removed. Consider also that some pain does not even originate from where we feel the hurt. Pain messages arising from local areas, and travelling along nerves to the spine and from there to the brain, can be re-routed, so that the pain is felt somewhere else altogether. This is known as reflex, or referred, pain (see pages 18–20). For example, angina pain is felt in the left arm (and other areas) but derives from distress in heart muscles.

Pain can be acute or chronic. Acute pain derives from a condition that builds rapidly to a crisis, such as a sprained ankle, whereas chronic pain is longer-lasting and more deep-seated – for example, back pain resulting from poor posture over a long period.

The way we experience most pain is affected not merely by the physical processes that have caused it to occur, but also by our intellectual and emotional reaction to it. Much depends on the "meaning" that we give the pain, which we tend to process through our individual experiences and expectations. Take, again, the arm pain of angina, which is similar to arm pain originating from hypersensitive areas of the muscles of the front of the neck (the scalenes). Your attitude toward the pain would be very different if you thought it were a neck-muscle problem, rather than a heart problem. What pain means to us, and the circumstances out of which it emerges, can radically affect our perception of its potency.

MEASURING YOUR PAIN

Pain is a personal experience – as difficult to measure and express objectively as hunger or thirst, happiness or sadness. You cannot say exactly *how much* a pain hurts, only that it is, for example, mild, moderate, severe or agonizing. However, your idea of what constitutes an "agonizing pain" may be very different from someone else's.

You can use the calibrated line shown below as a template to incorporate in a "pain journal" in which you record aspects of your pain experience (see pages 36–9). By marking your pain level on such a scale each day, you can keep a check on how your pain is changing over time, perhaps in response to different treatments or changes in behaviour (such as exercise or diet).

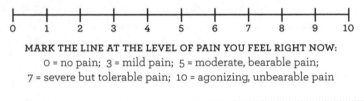

MARK THE LINE AT THE LEVEL OF PAIN YOU FEEL RIGHT NOW:
0 = no pain; 3 = mild pain; 5 = moderate, bearable pain;
7 = severe but tolerable pain; 10 = agonizing, unbearable pain

If we understand the cause of our pain, we are more likely to react to it in a constructive way.

Pain is sometimes positively useful. If you injure your arm, you know why it hurts afterwards. Days later the area may still be red and painful owing to the inflammatory process, without which the tissues could not heal (see pages 32–3). These healing tissues need to be treated with care so that they remodel themselves properly – the continued hurt is a warning to avoid doing too much too soon.

Sometimes, however, the cause of a pain is not clear, calling for expert investigation. In some cases, the original cause may be gone but its effects live on in a constant discomfort or worse. This occurs in conditions such as shingles (herpes zoster), after which burning pain can continue for years, serving no warning purpose at all. If you don't know why something hurts, you need to find out.

THE PAIN EXPERIENCE

What we think about pain, the meaning we give to it and the emotions we attach to it – such as unfounded fear, anxiety or apprehension – have major effects on our overall experience of pain. Recognizing that pain is both a signal-and-response process and an emotional, psychological experience can help us to manage it more effectively.

People can often learn to cope with even severe pain if challenged to do so, or if the circumstances in which the pain occurs demand that they ignore it. For example, we are more tolerant of productive pain

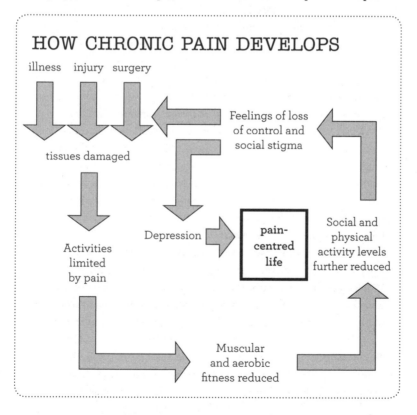

HOW CHRONIC PAIN DEVELOPS

illness injury surgery

tissues damaged

Feelings of loss of control and social stigma

Activities limited by pain

Depression

pain-centred life

Social and physical activity levels further reduced

Muscular and aerobic fitness reduced

(such as that associated with childbirth or life-enhancing surgery) than pain deriving from an accident. If we have difficulty coming to terms with pain, we risk developing "pain behaviour" (see also box, page 49). This involves over-compensating, for example by avoiding everyday tasks, such as getting dressed or preparing meals, or by performing them more slowly and with unnecessary caution.

Another factor that seems to influence how we respond to pain – even extreme pain – is our cultural background. Research has demonstrated that people from different cultures often respond to the same amount of pain in very different ways.

Work by Drs Ronald Melzack and Patrick D. Wall – perhaps the world's leading pain researchers – shows that when painful electric shocks are given to sensitive areas of the body, the level at which they are reported as "intolerable" varies widely, depending on the cultural background of the volunteers being tested. In one study, for example, Nepalese volunteers reported severe pain only when receiving a far higher level of electrical stimulation than European volunteers.

In another experiment, Melzack and Wall demonstrated that people could be challenged to increase their tolerance of the pain of holding a hand in icy water, if they were told that another person had been able to keep a hand in the water for longer than they had. This type of research suggests that we possess abilities to alter our pain tolerance through the power of suggestion, which has implications for how we can improve our handling of pain.

Research also suggests that our gender and "personality type" can have a bearing on the way in which we deal with painful conditions. Women handle pain better than men do, but consult a doctor about it more readily; and laid-back, calm people seem better able to cope with quite severe pain, compared to those who are nervous and anxious.

There is, therefore, an accumulation of evidence relating to "mind control" over pain. By observing the varying ways in which different people experience similar types of pain, researchers have been able to develop tactics to help people to manage their pain

SHUTTING THE PAIN GATE

Touching, rubbing or pressing an area of the body transmits sensations toward the spinal cord and brain along nerve pathways that are thicker than the thin fibres used to transmit pain impulses. These milder messages, which travel more quickly and therefore reach the brain sooner than pain messages, are produced by very low-threshold nerve endings (mechanoreceptors), which are far more easily activated than pain receptors. We therefore appear to be able to reduce the intensity of pain messages by modifying signals coming from a painful area with gentle stimulation, such as vibration or rubbing – this is called "shutting the pain gate".

Understanding how the pain gate mechanism can partially modify pain helps to explain the effectiveness of numerous therapies such as massage, acupressure and acupuncture. TENS (transcutaneous electrical nerve stimulation) machines have a similar pain-blocking effect – they work by passing a very mild electrical current across painful regions.

Not only do these therapies "shut the pain gate", but they also induce the body to release natural painkilling hormones that can further suppress pain signals. A combination of mechanical signals, self-produced hormones and thoughts and emotion can therefore interact to modify the degree of pain we experience.

better and sometimes even to overcome it completely. The science of cognitive behavioural therapy (CBT) has grown out of this research and forms a major part of the work of dedicated pain clinics. Managing pain means finding ways of living with it, so it does not dominate everyday activities, or prevent a fulfilling and active life. Many of these strategies are discussed in more detail later in this book. They include relaxation, meditation and visualization methods (see pages 60–84), hydrotherapy (see pages 119–21), and techniques that put the "gate theory" of pain into practice (see box, above).

MEET THE NERVOUS SYSTEM

"Pain is in the brain" – not where you feel the pain – so it's not always easy to know where pain messages are coming from. Sometimes it's pretty obvious – if, say, you stub your toe or bump your head. But often the pain you feel in one place originates somewhere else. Your experience of pain combines messages received and managed by your nervous system – involving conscious and unconscious processes – with your responses to the pain, such as changes in your posture, behaviour or function. To better understand pain we need to take a closer look at the nervous system.

The brain and the spinal cord form the central nervous system (CNS) and this receives messages from the peripheral nervous system (PNS), made up of nerves that feel (sensory) and those that activate (motor). Those aspects of the body over which we have little or no conscious control are governed by the autonomic nervous system (ANS), and this is itself divided into the sympathetic and the parasympathetic branches, which respectively stimulate or moderate functions such as the rate at which you breathe or your heart beats.

Within these systems and sub-systems are a host of "reflex pathways" that help manage the astonishingly intricate functioning of the body. It is along these pathways that messages such as pain are referred from one area to another. For example, viscero-somatic pathways carry pain that originates in an organ to a more mechanical part of the body, such as angina pain felt in the arm. Pain travelling in the opposite direction (along a somatico-visceral pathway) includes that felt in the heart, but caused by irritated nerve structures in the chest muscles. Messages can also be transmitted from one movable part of the body to another. A simple example is the defensive reflex that tells your arm to move your hand when you touch something hot.

Pain felt in a part of the body may even have an emotional, rather than a physical, cause. An example of this psychosomatic pain is the stomach ache you might feel before an exam.

In some cases, a single event can give rise to more than one pain message travelling along more than one pathway. For example, if you were to fall and twist your back, the vertebra that you twisted would be painful afterwards, but you might also suffer pain in one of your legs. This referred leg pain might be caused by the vertebra pressing onto a nerve; or you might have irritated some nerve structures in the joints connecting the vertebrae to each other; or you might have altered your posture to compensate for the initial pain in your back, thereby triggering pain in your leg; and of course memories of past experiences might colour the meaning you give to this back pain, and how you behave as a result.

CENTRAL AND PERIPHERAL NERVOUS SYSTEMS

AUTONOMIC NERVOUS SYSTEM

Parasympathetic nerves
Sympathetic nerves

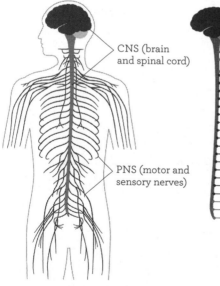

CNS (brain and spinal cord)

PNS (motor and sensory nerves)

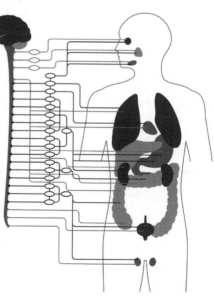

A remarkable aspect of all this confusion is that when researchers compare the progress of different back injuries of this sort, they find that, with or without treatment or medication, most of them are better within four weeks. The body usually heals itself. When it cannot, treatment is needed.

"Understanding pain physiology changes the way people think about pain, reduces its threat value and improves their management of it."

David Butler and Lorimer Moseley,

Explain Pain[1]

CENTRAL SENSITIZATION

To understand the origin of much chronic pain, it is essential to appreciate a process known as central sensitization. This may start when there are a number of peripheral (local) areas of constant or frequently recurring pain, possibly involving inflammation or infection.

When, despite appropriate treatment, a pain is constant or recurrent (happening over and over again with only short breaks in-between), and when there are simultaneously other recurrent or persistent areas of pain in the body, and when this continues for many months or years, the process of sensitization may start. The original peripheral pains might be musculoskeletal, such as neck, back, knee

THE PROCESS OF SENSITIZATION
Sensitization causes all pain to be perceived more strongly, and the area of pain to enlarge.

Dysfunction of pain-inhibiting nerve pathways in brain. The brain and central nervous system become sensitized, increasing perception of local/peripheral pain

Site of original injury

Dysfunction of pain-modulating descending nerve pathways

Overactive neural receptor sites at dorsal horn

Ascending nerve pathways overactive

Nociceptors in peripheral tissues become more sensitive

or elbow pains, and/or they might involve headache, toothache, stomach ache or discomfort affecting other organs (such as irritable bowel or painful bladder). Over time the sensitization process makes these pains more severe and wide-ranging – until the brain itself is sensitized and much of the body hurts most of the time.

As sensitization starts, changes occur to features of the pain:

- The nerves that register pain in the peripheral areas may become increasingly sensitive, so that their pain threshold is lowered and they report pain sensations more easily. This is known as hyperalgesia.

- With hyperalgesia peripheral nerves may start to report pain from a wider area, and these pain sensations may continue for longer than they originally did, so that a lesser stimulus produces a stronger and longer pain response.

- Pain may be reported with even extremely light stimuli that previously would not even have been sensed. This is known as hyperesthesia.

- Mild sensations, such as light pressure being applied, that would previously not have been painful, become painful. This is known as allodynia.

- Through a crossover of pain messages, sensations that were felt in an organ, say the stomach, become experienced in muscles, a process known as viscero-muscular hyperalgesia. Similar crossover pain can occur from organ to organ (known as viscero-visceral hyperalgesia).

- These changes can affect the actual function of organs – for example, leading to irritable bowel syndrome.

COMMON FEATURES IN PATIENTS DEVELOPING CENTRAL SENSITIZATION

In one study[2], 512 individuals with local back or neck pain were studied over a seven-year period to see how many would develop chronic widespread pain involving central sensitization, and to identify features shared by the group. It was found that 22.6 percent of those with local back or neck pain in 2001/2002 had developed central sensitization by 2007, and that six significant common features could be identified:

1   Pain was of moderate to severe intensity.

2   The majority were female.

3   There was a family history of chronic widespread pain, possibly due to genetic and/or familial environmental influences.

4   The individuals were mainly aerobically unfit as a result of their pain severely interfering with general activities of life, including exercise.

5   The majority displayed one or more central sensitivity syndromes, such as irritable bowel syndrome, irritable bladder syndrome, restless legs syndrome and/or migraines.

6   Numerous pain-management strategies were being used.

- Emotional and psychological consequences also result.

- When central sensitization is established, pain transmissions to the brain are exaggerated while, at the same time, the brain's normal pain-control methods are reduced. In a very real way, the brain itself becomes sensitized.

The end result of central sensitization can be seen in conditions such as fibromyalgia or myofascial pain syndrome, and in chronic migraine[3].

Recent research[4] has shown that, because the nervous system and the brain become sensitized, the associated features of this condition include hypersensitivity to many normal stimuli, such as bright light, touch, noise, pesticides, mechanical pressure, medication and high and/or low temperature.

Once central sensitization is established it may become self-perpetuating, even after the peripheral signals stop. However, there is increasing evidence that eliminating the peripheral triggers can reverse the sensitization process.

Other research[5] has shown that both local muscle pain – often caused by myofascial trigger points (see pages 99–101) – as well as joint pains can directly influence the development *and maintenance* of central sensitization, and that successful treatment of these local features reduces sensitization[6]. An understanding of central sensitization reinforces the need to deal appropriately and safely with minor, peripheral pains, rather than putting up with them.

" Take rest; a field that has rested gives a bountiful crop "

Ovid (43BCE–17CE)

CENTRAL HABITUATION

When the volume on a radio or TV is set too low, our brains interpret voices as background noise – we are unable to understand what is actually being said. In the same way, there is a threshold of stimulation below which nociceptors do not report pain to the brain.

As we have seen, sensitization can lead to extreme, widespread pain. However, the opposite outcome may also occur. If the prolonged or repeated irritation of pain receptors is only at a mild to moderate level, a process known as habituation might begin. With habituation, the reporting of pain to the brain actually reduces, rather than increasing as in central sensitization. More than just "getting used to the pain", habituation is a process in which the brain interprets non-threatening pain messages less strongly.

It seems that our perception of pain is the result of an interaction between pain-producing and pain-reducing mechanisms. Understanding how the nervous system responds to pain offers an opportunity to develop better treatment strategies. One study[7] has shown that when a group of healthy volunteers were given repeated painful experiences – for example, by having one of their arms exposed to 20 minutes of extreme cold, for eight consecutive days – the degree of pain reported (see page 14) reduced day by day, even though the same level of cold exposure was applied. The other arm and the legs also showed reduced sensitivity to the pain stimulus (in other words, they had also developed a higher tolerance to pain) – although not to the same extent as the originally tested arm.

> **TOP TIP** By making conscious relaxation a part of your daily routine, you can encourage a process of habituation to chronic pain that will help you manage your experience of it.

Interestingly, the higher pain tolerance persisted after the experiments were completed.

The researchers suggest that these changes in pain perception, which take place in the brain, probably represent a "defensive strategy against pain" by the brain. It is important to understand that the studies involved healthy adults and that similar habituation changes may not take place in the same way in individuals with existing chronic pain conditions – therefore research continues.

What we can learn from sensitization and habituation is that the amount of pain we feel, and how well we tolerate it, depends to a large extent on the way the brain interprets pain messages. The habituation response suggests that the brain and nervous system may be able to recognize when pain messages are of lesser importance. One objective in managing chronic pain might therefore be to encourage habituation, so that the brain can ignore unimportant pain messages. Methods such as relaxation and visualization, as well as recognizing pain for what it is without giving it excessive importance, appear to be ways of encouraging habituation. Whatever else we do about pain and its causes, we also need to try to reduce our overall stress levels, as these can have considerable influence on the pain load, and on sensitization to it.

THE STRESS EFFECT

Stress affects both the body and the mind. Stress is the body's reaction to a change – the stressor – that requires any physical, mental or emotional adjustment or response. Because stress can lead to, or aggravate, many forms of pain, we need to understand how it operates.

Stressors can be grouped into three main categories: biochemical (for example, dietary imbalances, infection, allergies and environmental pollution); biomechanical (over- or underuse of the body, poor posture and injuries); and psychosocial (emotional pressures, anxiety, fear, depression and so on). Combinations of such stressors affect all of us much of the time, and are usefully summarized as the "stress load".

We don't all handle our stress loads in the same way – how we cope depends on numerous factors including our inherited characteristics, culture, past experiences and beliefs. As we adapt to and manage (or fail to manage) the multiple stressors associated with modern life, we may reach a point when our adaptation begins to fail and health problems arise. When we reach our stress threshold, the self-repair processes of our mind and body stop adapting adequately to the multiple stresses. Like a strip of elastic stretched too far and for too long, adaptation is no longer possible and our health is damaged.

As the definition above suggests, stress is not always a response to negative factors, but can also be the by-product of positive, healthy changes to your lifestyle. For example, let's say that you take up fitness training. The first few exercise sessions will lead to stiffness and muscle soreness, but if you sustain your routine your body will adapt to the biomechanical stress by building new muscle fibres and improving your circulation to meet the raised oxygen demand.

More often, though, biomechanical stress results from sustained or repetitive inappropriate activity. If you sit slumped at a desk working a computer (or you play the guitar, dig the garden or drive a car) for too long, your body will adapt to the imposed stress by

THE THREE PHASES OF STRESS

The major researcher into stress (he was the first to use the word in this context) was the Hungarian-born scientist Hans Selye. He described typical phases of what he called the general adaptation syndrome as follows:

- An alarm phase occurs during which the body experiences an acute response to the stressor (known as a "fight-or-flight response").

- If the stressor is sustained, the body will go into a resistance phase, in which it will cope with the stressor (also described as adaptation or compensation).

- After prolonged exposure to that same stressor – or other stressors – the body's adaptive capacity fails and the exhaustion/collapse phase is reached, leading to dysfunction or disease.

EFFECT ON BODY OF PROLONGED STRESS

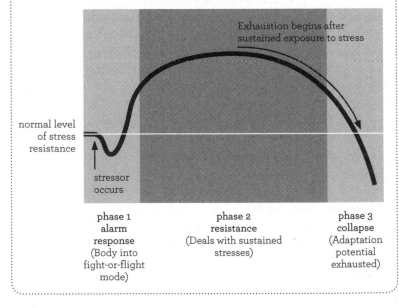

normal level of stress resistance

Exhaustion begins after sustained exposure to stress

stressor occurs

phase 1	phase 2	phase 3
alarm	resistance	collapse
response	(Deals with sustained	(Adaptation
(Body into	stresses)	potential
fight-or-flight		exhausted)
mode)		

tightening up overused muscles. Soon stiffness, local irritation or inflammation and, eventually, pain will develop. This form of biomechanical stress is often termed repetitive strain injury (see page 156).

What happens when stresses are multiple and excessive? Take someone whose work and leisure have created a physically and psychologically stressful lifestyle – insufficient rest time, inability to ease up, time pressures, repetitive or posturally uncomfortable activities, inadequate exercise. Add emotional stress relating to work, study, relationships or money, with sleep-pattern disturbances and a less-than-ideal diet, and an alarming picture emerges. Individually each of these stress factors may not cause a problem, but combined they can set the scene for pain and other adverse symptoms to develop. These symptoms then produce more stress as they, in turn, demand further adaptations from the body.

The good news is that just as a watch can be water proofed, so a person can – to a very large extent – be "stress proofed".

HELP YOUR BODY TO HELP ITSELF

The body has a built-in repair potential – an automatic tendency to restore its natural equilibrium (otherwise known as homeostasis). Normally, wounds heal, broken bones mend and infections clear. However, the efficiency with which homeostatic mechanisms do their work depends on your unique characteristics, both the ones you were born with and those you acquire through life, such as nutritional habits and posture.

The "staircase" diagram below shows examples of how life's multiple stresses (the stress load) can mount up to overwhelm your

SOME OF THE MULTIPLE STRESSORS OF LIFE

- Nutritional deficiencies
- Allergies, infections, inflammation
- Exposure to toxicity
- Abuse of drugs, nicotine, alcohol

- Acquired traits, such as previous and current ailments
- Personal hygiene
- Exercise and sleep factors – the habits of daily life

- Attention to hygiene, exercise, rest or sleep

- Your unique in-born (genetic) traits
- Learned behaviour

- Awareness of general health-maintenance behaviour

defence and repair systems, which leads to a situation known as heterostasis. When this happens we generally need outside help to restore homeostasis. We call that outside agency "treatment".

Our self-healing capability is enormous, and it is vital that we do not lose sight of this great gift. Our task when we are ill, or in pain, is to attempt to remove obstacles to recovery, to support and build up, as best we can, the multiple functions that make up homeostasis, and to avoid interfering with self-healing processes. The "staircase" diagram below shows some of the stresses that can escalate to overwhelm you. However, under the stairs are treatments to counter each of these stresses.

- Poor posture, poor breathing
- Over- and misuse of body
- Injuries, surgery
- Degenerative joint problems

- Appropriate exercise, stretching, Pilates, yoga, t'ai chi, physiotherapy, massage, osteopathy, acupuncture

- Stress levels (interpersonal, study, at work, financial)
- Anxiety, depression, anger
- Isolation, poor self-image

- Stress management, counselling, psychotherapy
- Breathing retraining, relaxation methods (such as meditation, visualization, autogenic training)
- Spiritual renewal, social support

- Reformed dietary habits, appropriate supplements, herbs, homeopathy, detox programmes
- Attention to possible pollutants at home and work

SOME OF THE TREATMENT AND SELF-HELP OPTIONS THAT CAN AID RECOVERY

INFLAMMATION IS GOOD FOR YOU

Inflammation is a natural and vitally important self-limiting process that helps the body repair and restore itself following damage, irritation and infection – our lives depend on it and, under normal circumstances, we "switch it off", by using anti-inflammatory medication, at our peril. However, at times inflammation can be excessive, with unacceptable levels of associated pain, and a degree of controlled inflammation reduction may be called for.

Our defence and repair mechanisms follow remarkable daily rhythms. The body systems that defend us from bacteria or viruses are far more active between roughly 10am and 10pm, leaving the night for tissue-repair processes involving inflammation. This explains why inflammation is often worse at night. Stressful events seem to alter these natural rhythms, so that the inflammatory phase may continue during the day. When this happens the defensive phase of the cycle is weakened, leaving the body more vulnerable to infection.

Over-the-counter, anti-inflammatory medicines, such as aspirin, should therefore be used with care, both because of their many potential side-effects (from stomach bleeding to severe liver and kidney problems) and because they often control inflammation *too* effectively. This slows down the repair of damaged tissues, causing you to use the area too soon and too much, worsening the problem.

There are a number of safe, natural methods for easing painful inflammation available as an alternative to medication. We can gently ease inflammation (and related pain) with diet, cutting down our intake of animal fats and increasing our intake of fish oils. This is helpful because animal fats contain large amounts of arachidonic acid, from which pro-inflammatory substances in the body – cytokines – are derived; whereas oily fish, such as sardines, salmon and tuna, contain high levels of eicosapentenoic acid (EPA), which studies have shown to counteract inflammatory activity. (See pages 128–32 for more anti-inflammatory dietary strategies.) Moderating stress levels can also help. We have seen that stress can interfere with defence-and-repair rhythms – by reducing stress we can reset the body's daily pattern. In addition, high levels of cortisol – the "stress hormone" – are linked to the release of cytokines. Reduced stress leads to reduced cortisol, and therefore moderation of these inflammatory chemicals.

CAUSES OF INFLAMMATION

Increased blood flow brings plasma and white blood cells to the damaged area, causing redness, heat, swelling and pain.

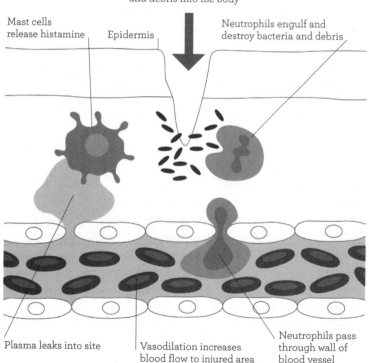

Injury introduces bacteria
and debris into the body

Mast cells
release histamine

Epidermis

Neutrophils engulf and
destroy bacteria and debris

Plasma leaks into site

Vasodilation increases
blood flow to injured area

Neutrophils pass
through wall of
blood vessel

THE PATH TO RECOVERY

The good news is that there are many ways in which we can manage most types of pain, and many of the conditions that cause them. Some of these pain-management techniques can be self-applied – and a selection of these are described in this book. Other treatments may need to be administered by conventional or complementary healthcare providers.

At this point it is important to emphasize, and to re-emphasize, that pain should never be ignored or masked with painkillers (see box, opposite) without you first understanding its cause. Remember also that any treatment needs to be both safe and to work with, rather than against, the body's self-repair mechanisms (see pages 30–31). It should not produce new symptoms!

Self-repair is not always possible – for example, in cases where pain is caused by chronic, degenerative conditions, such as osteoarthritis – so be realistic and reasonable in your expectations for improvement. In severe cases, methods used to control pain may need to be extreme, possibly involving drugs that carry side-effects, or surgery. However, even in such situations the general principles and specific therapies presented in this book can be used to complement those methods, helping to make life more tolerable.

Probably the most important factor governing how fast you travel the path toward improvement and recovery is your attitude and the way you make use of your inner reserve of strength – a store that we all have within us. Try to think constructively about your pain and be proactive in the recovery process. Tackling the management of your pain in a positive way should encourage you to take control of other aspects of your life. In this way your painful ordeal can provide an opportunity for reflection and change, enabling you to transform your lifestyle in ways you may often have considered, but never had the impetus to follow through.

OVER-THE-COUNTER PAIN KILLERS

Many medical methods set out to attack symptoms rather than treating causes, and a lesson we seem to have taken from that approach is "if it hurts, kill the pain", and if it's inflamed, deactivate the inflammation (see pages 32–3). To be fair, most doctors recognize that this sort of approach is not ideal, as pain (sometimes) and inflammation (almost always) serve key roles in the body's defence and self-repair processes. The failure of patients to appreciate the danger of self-prescribing medication, as well as constant promotion by pharmaceutical companies and the ready availability of such medication without prescription from pharmacies and supermarkets, keeps the sales of painkillers and anti-inflammatories booming.

This is not to deny that at times such medication may be a useful first aid. But there are significant dangers in stopping pain before its message has been understood. For example, a painful knee may signal the onset of an easily managed cartilage problem. However, if the sufferer takes painkillers, then uses the knee in running, jumping or even walking, the damage may worsen – sometimes irreparably.

Kill the pain and this is the possible outcome. Recognize the cause and the problem can usually be fixed – and the pain will go away.

It's worth repeating a comment made earlier in this chapter: When a fire alarm rings, finding the source of the fire is far more urgent than switching off the alarm.

KEEPING A PAIN JOURNAL

Can you recall how you felt at any given moment over the past week, and what you had to eat for each meal, and make connections between these factors and the degree of pain you experienced? Most people would find it difficult to recall these details, yet they contain valuable clues to the pattern and possible causes (or irritants) of your symptoms. It is useful to record such information in a journal or on a chart, to be analyzed by you or a healthcare professional.

Use the list of questions below, and the sample journal entry on the pages 38–9, as a basis for your own journal. Writing down the data also gives you a chance to analyze it. As you make regular entries, you may well notice patterns emerging in your activities and symptoms. By altering aspects of your daily life, you can manage your experience of pain.

QUESTIONS TO STRUCTURE YOUR PAIN JOURNAL:

- Is the pain constant or intermittent? If the latter, what pattern does it follow? Which activities increase or decrease the pain?
- Is the pain aching, burning, sharp, stabbing, cramp-like or tingling?
- Is there swelling, redness or heat in the area of pain?
- Does it still hurt when you rest, or does rest ease the pain?
- Is it easier when you move around? If so, what sort of movement eases it?
- Is the pain affected by certain foods and drinks? If so, which?
- Is the pain affected by emotional factors? If so, which?
- If you are female, is the pain affected by aspects of your menstrual cycle?

A journal (or part of it) can be specifically focused. For example, if there seems to be a link between a chronic pain and certain foods, try keeping a food journal with a symptom score sheet to assess the effects of including or excluding particular foods (see pages 135–40).

List everything you eat, as well as the times of day you have your meals. Record any variation in the pattern of your symptoms and try to note down the precise time at which the symptoms varied. (The example of a symptom score sheet below highlights the effects on pain of stress, Pilates, rest and massage.)

Your journal should give you room to describe your feelings in relation to your pain (as well as to life events) to see how these might be influencing each other. The journal offers a chance to explore

SYMPTOM SCORE SHEET

DATE	12 May	13 May	14 May	15 May	16 May	17 May
NECK PAIN	2	1	1	2	3	2
HEADACHE	2	1	1	3	3	2
FATIGUE	3	2	1	3	2	1
INDIGESTION	1	0	0	2	1	0
SLEEP	1	2	0	2	1	1
CONCENTRATION	2	3	1	2	1	1
TOTAL	11	9	4	14	11	7
notes	Started Pilates class	Ached post Pilates but felt looser	Good day! Chinese meal	Stressful day at work	No desk work – rested	Pilates class + massage

Every day at the same time of the day score each symptom
for the previous 24 hours:
3 = worst possible; 2 = moderately bad; 1 = mild; 0 = no problem

anger, fear, anxiety or any other strong emotions, perhaps with the help of someone else. Be careful to record information accurately in the journal, as regularly as you can, but don't become obsessive about it. It is simply something to aid your memory and help you to understand the bigger picture surrounding your pain.

The sample journal below has been used to set manageable daily targets for improved diet, flexibility and relaxation. On the left, the

PAIN JOURNAL

PAIN BAR

No pain   Extreme pain

Location
of pain

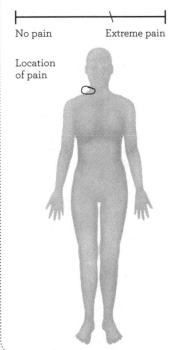

DATE July 25th

PHYSICAL SYMPTOMS

Ache (dull with sharp twinges) across top of shoulders. Hub deep within base of neck and either side of spine. Stiffness and headache later in day.

MENTAL SYMPTOMS

Extremely stressed! Couldn't think clearly and couldn't concentrate for more than a few minutes at a time.

EMOTIONAL SYMPTOMS

Fluctuating between feeling really sad and frustrated (because I couldn't complete things quickly) and irritability.

WHAT AGGRAVATES / EASES PAIN

Aggravates: sudden head movements, staring at computer for a long time. Eases: neck and shoulder rolls, brisk walk home from station, bath before bedtime.

intensity of pain is recorded on a "pain bar". A body map enables you to plot the pain's location or locations. A detailed plan including general lifestyle goals will help you gain more control over your life – and your pain. Make a separate column in your journal to record how successful you have been in achieving your aims.

PLAN	ACTUAL
DIET	
Drink: 2 litres water and eat 4 pieces fruit Breakfast: oats (skimmed milk) Lunch: tomato soup (with roll, no butter) Dinner: chicken and salad	All done! (except one snack of a biscuit at mid-afternoon)
MOVEMENT	
AM: 10 mins neck rolls and shoulder rolls PM: 10 mins bicep stretches and back stretches and head and neck rolls	All done!
RELAXATION	
10 minute visualized meditation before bed 5 minutes breathing (any time)	Missed the breathing – schedule in more firmly for tomorrow
GOALS	
* Leave work on time (to increase relaxation time) * Call a friend (to keep in touch)	Left 15 minutes late – an improvement Called Anne – it was great to talk to her, she's doing really well!

POSITIVE ATTITUDES

Our personal response to chronic pain can vary widely. For some, the problem of pain may be a challenge to be managed practically, while for others it might be a looming threat beyond their influence – a burden to be endured.

"Hardiness" is a term used in psychology to describe a group of traits that, when they are strongly present in a person's way of coping with life, make for more positive approaches and healthier outcomes. Hardiness can also be gauged by the presence of a sense of control, that life's challenges can be overcome, and by what has been described as mental flexibility. There are a number of variations between these extremes, with positive and negative attitudes to pain varying over time.

The good news is that it is possible to develop hardiness traits, and to see favourable results emerging from even the darkest of situations.

TURNING THE MENTAL KEY

While it may seem counter-intuitive to suggest that health problems, with chronic pain as a prime example, can offer positive, life-enhancing opportunities, this does seem to be the case for some individuals, and it may be possible to draw lessons from such examples. A group of helpful positive characteristics have been identified as invaluable in facing up to painful and threatening conditions – together these are described as the "hardiness factor" (or "resilience factor"). Hardiness in this sense comprises the presence of three main attributes, summarized as challenge, control and commitment. These features have been studied in many pain-related settings – for example in people with fibromyalgia[1] as well as in painful AIDS-related diseases[2].

CHALLENGE

Stress and the problems of life, including chronic pain, may be viewed as challenges that can be overcome if they are properly understood. People who see stress or chronic pain in this light are likely to be motivated to address causes in positive ways that give a sense of purpose and meaning to life. Contrast this approach with one in which stress and chronic pain are viewed as overwhelming forces that crush, rather than motivate. Research has suggested that by making a conscious effort to view life more optimistically, your expectations and behaviour will change accordingly, resulting in more positive outcomes than you had previously imagined possible.

CONTROL

This attribute is defined as the extent to which an individual feels a sense of autonomy and an ability to influence (if not fully control) life for the better, as it unfolds. A person with control feels that even when true mastery of a challenge is not possible, whatever possibilities do exist can and should be explored. Many people who experience pain (and even those who don't) have feelings of powerlessness, of being at the mercy of fate. When you begin to exercise control over aspects of your pain, you take the first step toward empowerment, even if the control you exercise over your pain is only temporary and partial. An example might be something as simple as booking an acupuncture session or taking up yoga.

COMMITMENT

People who have hardiness characteristics feel that their life has purpose (whatever shape that may take), and this purpose motivates them to try actively to shape their surroundings and to persevere even when their attempts to influence life don't appear to be working out. In contrast a person who has no motivation, and no commitment, will be less likely to lead a resilient, committed life in which they find meaning in their activities even though faced with significant adversity such as pain. Chronic pain can make it all too easy to withdraw from other people, to avoid social contact, to become isolated. But to a large extent this is a choice we make for ourselves, and as with all choices there are other possible options.

The media frequently portrays individuals who have suffered enormously, yet have overcome the vicissitudes of their lives to become beacons of hope and examples to us all. These are people who, despite being crippled by injury or born with major disabilities, have set aside their scars and pain and made a positive contribution. Some of these people may have inborn personality traits that help them achieve this degree of commitment, but they are also choosing to exercise these traits and are refusing to be beaten by circumstances. Research shows that commitment is greatly helped by a strong social support system, whether this involves friends, family, a partner or professional advisers (see box, page 45). Even if you feel that you are alone, there are always people to whom you can turn. Choosing to ignore those who can offer support can add to feelings of isolation.

There are a number of ways in which you can engage with other people. Try speaking to someone frankly, uncomplainingly, about your pain, so that they (and you) come to a clearer understanding of your problems. Or you could join a self-help group, where people in a similar situation support each other and discuss shared issues. Another option might be to identify someone in need and to do what *you* can to help *them*. In this way you will not only benefit someone else, but also force yourself to look beyond your own suffering.

Many of the ideas and exercises outlined in later pages of this book offer ways of enhancing hardiness.

" Nothing has any power over me,
other than that which I give it
through my conscious thoughts. "

Anthony Robbins (b. 1960)

UNLOCK YOUR POTENTIAL

There is no shortcut to exercising control, to reducing your sense of isolation or to viewing problems as challenges rather than threats. This exercise will help you to take the first steps – the most important and most difficult – toward strengthening those aspects of hardiness that may not currently be strong features of your personality, or toward enhancing them if they already are. As you find yourself becoming more and more confident in these three techniques, they should become second nature, so that they begin to influence your way of approaching all aspects of life.

1   To foster a sense of control, start by identifying a treatment or therapy that is likely to help your pain. Write a list of steps that you need to take – say, making appointments or buying equipment – to make your project take shape. Set yourself target dates for each step. If you give your plan structure by writing it down, you will have a tangible starting point, rather than just a mass of good intentions in your head.

2   To avoid cutting yourself off from the outside world, call a friend at least once a week. Make sure that you don't talk just about your pain, but also discuss what is happening to your friend. Arrange to meet them when you feel ready – but don't rush yourself.

3   To help you to view obstacles as challenges, transform your negative statements into positive ones. Train yourself to stop in your tracks when you find yourself saying something like, "I don't stand a chance." Revise your statement and say it aloud – for example, "Although it may be difficult, I can do it." Affirmations of this sort can be helpful in creating a more positive attitude – aim to see the glass half full, rather than half empty.

FAMILY RESILIENCE

Chronic pain is seldom life-threatening, but is marked by its lengthy duration (at least six months to qualify for the designation "chronic") or frequent recurrence over a long period. There may be a slow progression of severity, persisting over time, with no easily definable beginning, middle or end. Chronic pain has the potential to negatively affect a person's family relationships, emotional well-being, friendships, occupation and leisure time – as well as having a direct financial impact. The solitary experience of chronic pain can diminish a person's role within the family physically, emotionally and psychologically, and often results in a reduced sense of self-worth as sufferers reduce their activities to focus on their physical state, experiencing multiple vague symptoms.[3]

The idea of "family resilience" (or hardiness), as a means of managing chronic pain, highlights the potential for family, relationship or social support in this process. Although the application of this model of care may involve professionals – such as nurses or health visitors – it is not difficult to see how its basic principles can be adapted to self-application.[4] The key feature is identifying and building on perceived relationship strengths (see list opposite), rather than focusing on deficits, encouraging greater resourcefulness in facing immediate and long-term challenges.

The successful ability of a family (or couple or social group) not just to cope with, but to weather crises together and emerge stronger and more resourceful, is the basis of family resilience. This approach focuses on the influence of positive relationships between people.

Research indicates that all families have strengths, and that by building on these the adverse effects of chronic pain can be reduced. This approach supports the re-establishment, or reinforcement, of communication between family members (or couples) and, by placing an emphasis on strengths, helps to shift the focus away from the problem of pain. A family resilience model of chronic pain

IDEAL FAMILY RESILIENCE CHARACTERISTICS

Your task is to identify which of the main family resilience (hardiness) attributes and resources you can draw on, and to encourage and work with these. Aim to develop those that aren't present, perhaps using some of the varied exercises and suggestions outlined later in this book.

- A positive outlook: sense of humour, confidence, optimism. Spirituality: values that are shared with others that may offer meaning to the situation, the stressors and the pain.

- Accord: avoidance of conflict; a sense of cohesion.

- Flexibility: the ability to adjust and modify family or relationship roles depending on circumstances.

- Communication: the ability to express feelings and emotions openly; collaborative problem solving – "you are not alone".

- Financial considerations: maintaining family warmth, despite possible economic pressures.

- Mutual family/relationship time

- Shared recreation

- Routines and rituals: the personal, private, internal activities of couples and families that can be encouraged in order to promote closer relationships.

- External support: networks of condition-specific contacts, shared resources, internet chatrooms, social networking websites.

management does not suggest that people will always "bounce back", untouched by their experiences; rather it proposes focusing on what works, instead of just looking at their problems.[5]

MIND OVER MATTER

Someone who is handed an ice cube under hypnosis, and told that it is intensely hot, will feel burning and drop it. They may even develop a blister in response to its "heat". The mind controls what we feel, and if the mind is persuaded that there is danger (even if, in reality, there is none) it will defend the body in a way it deems appropriate (a blister is a protective response to a burn). What the mind believes determines the meaning of pain – and there are ways of safely modifying beliefs that may have been reinforcing pain, rather than modifying it.

Extreme examples can be seen in people who suffer injuries, such as torn muscles when playing sport, and feel no pain at the time. They disassociate themselves from the pain – it is unimportant in the context of the intense emotions of the event. If it is possible for the mind to delete or modify pain in this way, it should also be possible to learn to apply such techniques consciously, and so to exercise the benefits of mind-control in the management of pain.

Hypnosis uses techniques that may be able to help you change the way you perceive your pain (other methods include biofeedback, see page 61, and visualization, see pages 81–4). A hypnotherapist will help you to construct a "script" to modify beliefs and feelings that are hampering you. (As a first step, you may rename your pain as "discomfort", for example.) Having guided you into deep relaxation, the therapist will recite the script to you. It might include something like: "See your discomfort – it has a size and a shape. Watch it change shape, get smaller, lighter. Feel its effect on you getting less and less." You can also record the script onto a CD or smartphone and practise self-hypnosis in this way.

PAIN BEHAVIOUR

The power of the mind is so strong that it can modify your behaviour in potentially harmful ways. For example, if you believe that the pain in your body represents a threat to life itself, or that it is likely to result in serious disability, you will tend to behave in ways that protect you from feeling the pain, but which will as a result prevent you from functioning normally, with negative consequences.

Being careful, avoiding aggravation of the condition or the pain, is one thing, but it is quite another to become ultra-cautious – to allow what is known as "pain behaviour" to dominate your life. Pain-avoidance behaviour, in which you avoid everyday activities "just in case" they upset the painful condition, can swiftly lead to you becoming so out of condition that normal activity is ever more difficult. It may even be that your focus on the pain is so great that it limits your belief in the possibility of recovery. Thankfully there are ways to modify such behaviour and beliefs:

- Learn more about your condition, and see that it may actually be made worse by inactivity (see pages 107–111), so that accurate information – rather than fear – allows you to alter your attitude.
- Start to become active in the self-management of your pain, your emotions and your environment, and develop a structured plan to gradually increase your levels of activity, with broadening horizons rather than shrinking ones – so that you modify behaviour patterns that may be holding back improvements that are within reach.

To get back on the road to "wellness behaviour", try making a list of pleasurable activities that you now avoid doing because of your pain. Think about which ones it may be possible to take up again and write down how you are going to achieve your aims. Make a start on at least one item within the next 24 hours.

AFFIRMATIONS

When pain is severe, prolonged feelings of despair and helplessness can be overwhelming. Used with confidence in their effectiveness, affirmations – repeated positive statements – can bolster your determination to overcome the enslavement of pain, promoting a positive balance to dominant negativity.

The pairs of statements shown on the next page are just examples, on which you may or may not choose to base your own affirmations. When constructing your own statements try to ensure that you do not use any negative or hesitant language.

For example, "I can achieve any ambition I set my mind to. I am positive and assured" is far more helpful than "I might be able to achieve my ambitions if I try. I am not negative or lacking assurance."

A key word in deciding to use affirmations is "choice". Choosing to listen to the advice of those who advocate affirmation tactics is, in itself, affirmative action. Of course, to have doubts about the validity of such claims is perfectly understandable. However, when there's an obvious need to create a positive sense of purpose in the face of a painful condition, scepticism about a process that can patently do no harm, and that might help, is self-limiting. Put aside your reservations and approach affirmations as though they were unquestionably valuable. Try them regularly, as often as you can, especially when you are feeling down. Make it your goal to prove that they really do work.

- Say these affirmations *every day, more than once,* even before you believe them.

- Say them as you look at yourself in the mirror, with conviction and ideally with a smile.

- Say them in the *present tense.*

When pain makes you anxious and tense
"My body and mind bathe in the light of the spirit."
"I let go of my worries. I am free to reach my goals."

When pain brings depression
"My pain is a fraction of my life. My fulfilment is infinitely larger."
"My life is still under my control. My self, and my relationships, are whole."

When pain returns
"The body follows its own wisdom. Healing continues."
"Even summer skies have clouds. I have come through before."

When pain makes you irritable
"No one is responsible for my pain. I will reach out to everyone I value."
"I am a calm pool, endlessly fed by the love of family and friends."

When pain makes you feel isolated
"Others hold me in their love, even when they are absent."
"My contribution is undiminished, even when I need to rest."

When pain is linked to past events
"I lovingly release the past — it is free and I am free."
"All is well in my heart. My pain is melting away."

When pain requires great strength
"I have the will to overcome my pain, to live as fully as I can."
"I can achieve anything I set my mind to. I am positive and assured."

When pain accompanies feelings of fear
"I breathe in the feeling of being calm and peaceful; I breathe out fear."
"My body is calm and peaceful, and my [body part] pain is healing."

MAKING IT HAPPEN

Good intentions are rarely enough. How well do you follow a plan or take health advice? The truth is that even when we are well and free from pain, every single one of us could make a list of things we ought to be doing (or ought to stop doing) that would almost certainly make us healthier, now or in the long run. And there have undoubtedly been times when you have ignored some of the sound, health-enhancing advice given to you by your doctor.

This is human nature – so it's worth being aware of the potential pitfalls as you start to make plans for your recovery from pain, to avoid weighing yourself down with blame or guilt when you fail to do everything you set out to accomplish. It's all too easy to give up when you find yourself not quite able or willing to do all that's needed. By anticipating at the outset the possibility of difficult periods, lapses or partial failure, you are less likely to abandon your plan completely.

Reducing the mechanical, chemical and psychological stresses on your body will always lead to better functioning of your repair and regeneration systems (see pages 27–9). As you see initial improvements in your experience of pain, your motivation to continue with your plan should get stronger. Unfortunately, though, the chances are that your motivation will plateau and begin to tail off when you reach a marked reduction in your pain. To ward off complacency, you may need to freshen up your strategy by regularly re-evaluating your goals and the methods you use to achieve them (see page 168). Reviewing your pain journal (see pages 36–9) on a regular basis will enable you not only to build up an understanding of your condition, to set your goals and monitor your success in achieving them, but also to identify new directions to take.

Motivation involves a desire to change things for the better and requires a belief that the changes you are asking yourself to make can indeed bring about an improvement. Your belief should be based on realistic objectives, not false hopes, which is why you should gather information and understand the whys and wherefores of whatever changes you are making. Armed with this knowledge, you will be making a conscious choice to take the path to wellness and recovery.

An obvious and appropriate place to start your fact-finding mission is your doctor. Traditionally, the relationship between patient and doctor has been an unequal one – the doctor gives instructions for you to follow, even if you don't fully understand the reasoning behind the treatment. However, it may be more constructive to think of the doctor–patient relationship as a partnership, in which the patient actively agrees to a course of action having understood the rationale behind it. Studies suggest that the better we understand why we are expected to exercise, alter our diet or apply relaxation methods, and so on, the more likely we are to find the motivation to persist with the treatment. Many good treatment or self-help plans do not succeed because of our failure to stick to the task. In medical terms this is known as failure to adhere to or comply with the plan, advice or prescribed approach – and is just as common when following advice from others as it is when acting on your own research.

If you want your plans to become a reality, it is important to set yourself appropriate, attainable targets. You can help yourself by following these steps:

- Understand the physiology of your pain problem, so you have a clear idea of how you can modify it (see pages 55–6 on enhancing compliance strategies).
- Practise visualizing the pain-generating processes, so that you can more effectively generate mental images that positively influence the situation.
- Develop and practise methods and exercises that enhance pain reduction and improve function.
- Allow time for these elements to work together to produce results – and to do so you need to stick to your plan, with periodic reviews of progress (using your pain journal as a tool).

PERSONAL RESOURCES

Health psychologists have identified four personality areas, known as our "personal resources", which have a significant impact on how well motivated we are likely to be in applying self-help strategies:

- **Body awareness** describes your ability to focus on different parts of your body in turn and to understand the needs of each – practising the autogenic training exercise on page 64 will help to improve your body awareness.

- **Self-focus** involves accepting yourself and your needs, being able to take care of yourself and having a sense of your own value. Visualizations (see pages 81–4) and affirmations (see pages 50–51) can encourage these qualities.

- **Locus of control** depends on whether you see events as being out of your control, or whether you believe you can influence them (see pages 44–4). You can learn to move your locus from beyond you to within you.

- **Coping ability** involves recognizing your current limitations and working within them. Someone with little coping ability is liable to ignore their pain and overdo things, causing a setback in their recovery. The information and exercises in this book should greatly improve your coping abilities so that you can apply self-knowledge in the choices you make each day.

ENHANCING COMPLIANCE

If, as the evidence suggests, understanding your pain is essential to dealing with it, the way you absorb information is also of some importance. The strategies that you choose to improve the efficiency of your pain-modifying techniques[6] will depend on whether you are an auditory, visual or kinesthetic learner. Are you someone who learns and understands by hearing information? Or are you someone who is more likely to retain information if you read about it? Or do you learn by being physically active – and best retain the essence of written material if it is presented in a lively and colourful manner?

If you know which of the descriptions most accurately applies to you, you can work to your strengths when learning about, planning and carrying out strategies to reduce pain.

If you are an auditory learner:

- Use verbal communication with others, and with yourself if need be, possibly recording information and affirmations so that you can play these back.
- Consider repeating information out loud to yourself, over and over again.
- Keep the messages simple, snappy and if possible rhythmic.

If you are a visual learner:

- Use written and visually stimulating illustrated material to inform yourself.
- Create mental pictures that you can refer to – particularly in visualization exercises (see pages 82 and 84).
- Use computers for accessing and displaying material and consider making use of their sound dimension as well.

If you are a kinesthetic learner – who learns by "doing":

- Try the physical exercises described later in the book (see the "Bodywork and Rehabilitation" and "Complementary Therapies" chapters in particular).
- Try to ensure as far as possible that information is presented to you in ways that support this approach to learning – reinforcing retention of ideas by tying them to physical movements, for example. So if you are reading instructions for an exercise (such as one for a better breathing pattern), you should actually perform the exercise at the same time – ideally while someone else evaluates how well you are following the steps.

" A journey of a thousand miles must begin with a single step. "

Lao-Tzu (604–531 BCE)

PROBLEM SOLVING

It is all too easy to slip into the habit of avoiding everyday tasks that your pain makes difficult. This exercise will help you to work out – and to carry out – plans to make these activities more manageable.

1   Write down a list of any activities of daily life that you find awkward because of your pain. These could include getting dressed, cooking, going shopping or doing something specific at work, such as sitting at a computer.

2   Choose one of your problem areas. Give it a "difficulty score" from 0 to 10, where not being able to do it at all would be worth 10, and being able to do it perfectly and painlessly would be worth 0. What's the "value" of this difficult task right now?

3   Now, make a list of strategies: any tactics, equipment, assistance, training or relearning of skills that might help you to achieve the difficult task more easily.

4   Assess your list of strategies. Which are the easiest ones to do? Do them first. Do any of them require outside help? Get it. Are they things you can organize for yourself? Do so. Start to put your plan into action - today.

5   Repeat Steps 2–4 for each of the items on your original list of problem areas. Record each activity in your pain journal.

6   Each week score the activities again in your pain journal – watch the total values drop as your plans take shape.

FINDING
PEACE

Picture yourself calm and pain-free. In the previous chapter you saw how it is possible to use the power of the mind to begin to feel this way. This chapter brings you tried-and-tested methods designed to guide you toward what is known as the "relaxation response". This is the exact opposite of the "stress response" (in which we tense ourselves and withdraw from painful situations).

The many ways in which relaxation can be achieved differ from person to person. For some, it might involve physical tensing and releasing of muscles, to "remind" the body what it feels like to "let go". For others, breathing, meditation or visualization exercises may be more effective. Try a range of the techniques presented here and practise those that work best for you. By repeated application you should see heartening improvements emerging over the coming weeks.

RELEASE YOUR MUSCLES TO RELEASE YOUR MIND

When you experience constant or repetitive pain, or are anxious in any way, your muscles become tense, preventing easy relaxation. This inability to relax physically can create a vicious circle of ever-increasing tension, fatigue, anxiety and pain. Fortunately, there are many techniques that will allow you to both prevent and counteract the effects of excessive physical tension.

Tense muscles require more oxygen than relaxed ones, but the irony is that the blood vessels that carry fresh, oxygenated blood into the muscle are constricted by the tightened tissue. This situation is aggravated by shallow breathing, something that is likely to happen when you are anxious, and if you have neglected physical (aerobic) activity (see page 66). Also, when muscles are tense, waste products

SOME EFFECTS OF FIGHT OR FLIGHT
A range of physiological changes occur
in response to perceived threat.

pupils dilate

mouth dries

adrenal glands release
adrenaline (to raise heart
rate, etc) and cortisol (to
depress immune system)

liver releases glucose
(to provide energy
for movement)

digestion slows or halts

muscles tense
(ready for action)

brain gets body into
action mode

palpitations occur

heart rate increases

breathing becomes
faster and more
shallow (to increase
flow of oxygen to
muscles)

blood pressure rises

sphincters relax

BIOFEEDBACK

Biofeedback can enable you to alter aspects of the way your body functions – warming or relaxing areas, for example – just by thinking about them. As chronic pain is usually accompanied by distressing emotional feelings, it's useful to realize that our emotions influence nerve-related chemicals that directly affect the intensity of pain – and also that biofeedback can help you change both emotions and pain.[1]

A biofeedback device for use at home is usually small and relatively inexpensive, with electrodes that measure aspects of body function, such as your pulse or breathing rate, or how tense or warm an area is. The device then feeds this information back to you as a screen image or sound, such as a flashing light or bleep for every heartbeat. Examples of how biofeedback works include:

- Measuring muscle tension in the painful area. Most people can feel changes in muscle tension (see the exercise on page 63). You can learn how to reduce muscle tension (and therefore pain) using changes in the sound or the image as a guide.

- Monitoring local temperature of the affected tissues, using the device to learn, through instructions sent to that body part from your brain, to increase or decrease the temperature.

- Measuring changes in your breathing rate – something that is directly linked to your emotional state (see page 66).

By relaxing deeply and focusing on the biofeedback machine and the function being measured, you can train yourself (virtually by trial and error) to increase or reduce the interval between the flashes or beeps, and by doing so alter body function, such as your blood pressure or heart rate. Initial instruction is usually necessary before practising on your own at home. Biofeedback has a high success rate in pain relief and is often used by physiotherapists and in specialized pain clinics.

drain away less efficiently. A combination of poor oxygenation of muscle tissue and retention of metabolic wastes lead to discomfort and stiffness – which creates even more tension! This tense state, known as "sympathetic arousal", is part of the fight-or-flight mechanism, originally intended to prepare you to run away from danger, or to defend yourself against it.

When the alarm is raised, adrenaline is released, which automatically causes your muscles to tense. At the same time your heart and breathing rate and blood pressure all increase to service the anticipated demands of the body. Many other instant-reflex events occur – these are all reversed as soon as the danger has passed. However, if there were an extended period of emergency, and alarm and stress continued, your muscles would stay permanently tense and you would remain constantly prepared for action. This prolonged state of sympathetic arousal is a recipe for exhaustion and pain.

In time, muscle tension can become habitual. This physical unease can feed back to the brain messages that you are anxious or agitated, taking you still further away from a state of relaxation. You may reach a point at which you are no longer even aware of how tense your muscles are, and releasing them becomes increasingly difficult. This means that if you try to relax, the effect will probably be the opposite – you may tighten your muscles even more, because you will have forgotten what relaxation feels like. In such a situation relaxation has to be relearned.

A word of caution is needed here. When someone who has not been able to relax for a long time finally achieves feelings of release, the first experiences of letting go can be almost frightening, as though they are losing control. So be prepared to feel slightly "lost" when you begin to relax. You are, however, perfectly safe – all that is happening is that you are undergoing a new (or old, but forgotten) set of sensations. Remember that everything that is happening as you relax is ultimately within your control. You can stop when you wish, restart when you wish, or even tense up again – if you wish.

PROGRESSIVE MUSCULAR RELAXATION

This exercise helps you to recognize muscular tension as it builds up, allowing you to stop it before it becomes locked in. It would be even more helpful if you were also using biofeedback (see page 61) that measured muscular tension. Results can come quickly if you do the exercise regularly. To derive the full progressive benefit, perform it every day for 5–10 minutes. Eventually you may find that you can release the tension of your muscles without first tensing them, simply by scanning the body and letting tension go (as in Step 5).

1   Lie on the floor, arms and legs outstretched. Clench the fist of your dominant hand for 10 seconds. Let go and enjoy the sense of release for 10–15 seconds. Repeat. Then repeat twice on your other hand.

2   Curl the toes of the foot on your dominant hand side upward toward the sky. Hold for 10 seconds. Release and relax for 10–15 seconds. Repeat, then repeat twice on the other foot.

3   Perform the same sequence in at least five other sites, or pairs of sites, working up from your feet to your head. For example: pull your kneecaps toward the hip to tense thigh muscles; squeeze your buttocks together; pull in your abdomen; hold a breath and at the same time draw your shoulder blades together; frown hard.

4   Practise daily for a few weeks. Then begin tensing and relaxing groups of muscles – all the muscles in the neck or chest, for example – and letting go to enjoy the sense of ease.

5   After another week, abandon the tension element – simply focus on the different regions and instruct tense areas to release and relax. This will be much easier if you also practise the exercise for autogenic training (see page 64).

AUTOGENIC TRAINING

There is now a great deal of evidence that autogenic training – "biofeedback without a machine" – can teach you to influence beneficially your autonomic nervous system. By following these steps for approximately 10 minutes each day you will learn to project certain sensations onto specific parts of your body, to relax muscles, improve circulation or relieve inflammation.

1   Lie comfortably, with a cushion under your head, your knees bent, feet flat on the floor and eyes closed. Focus on your dominant arm and silently say, "My arm feels heavy." Visualize and sense the arm relaxed and heavy. For about a minute repeat the affirmation, "My arm feels heavy." Your mind may wander periodically. Don't worry, this is normal – just return your attention to your arm and its heaviness. Enjoy the sense of release – of letting go – that comes with this feeling.

2   Next, focus on your other arm and do exactly the same thing for about a minute.

3   Now focus your attention on your left leg and then on your right leg, each time for about a minute. Repeat affirmations about the relaxed weight of your limbs all the while.

4   Return to your dominant arm and this time say to yourself, "My arm is feeling warm." Apply this warming message to your three other limbs in the same order as before, focusing on each for about a minute. Feel the warmth spread and enjoy this sensation.

5   Focus on your forehead and affirm that it feels cool and refreshed. Hold this thought for a minute or so. Finally, stretch: clench your fists, bend your elbows and extend your arms. Open your eyes feeling alert and relaxed.

It is crucial, though, that you do find a way to rid yourself of tension, because only with the onset of relaxation can your body reverse the damaging hormonal processes that stress induces. Bringing about these positive biochemical changes will dramatically reduce your pain levels.

As a first step toward liberating yourself from a state of tension you can use well-tried muscular relaxation exercise methods, the best known of which is called progressive muscular relaxation (see exercise, page 63). Other ways of releasing muscular tension, and so helping to calm the mind, include stretching methods (such as yoga and muscle energy technique, see pages 103–106) and biofeedback (see page 61).

Autogenic training, which combines elements of progressive muscular relaxation and meditation, works on the part of your nervous system that you can't usually control, known as the autonomic nervous system. This is divided into the sympathetic nervous system, which produces alarm sensations – such as the fight-or-flight response – and creates feelings of apprehension and anxiety; and the parasympathetic nervous system, which produces calming relaxation feelings (see pages 18–19). The autogenic training exercise opposite will help you to learn how to control some aspects of these autonomicresponses, easing the sympathetic and enhancing the parasympathetic.

In time, if you become well practised in the exercises in this section, you will reach a point where you will be able to recognize tension building up, and will automatically, without even doing the exercises, be able to "switch it off". For example, with autogenic training you will be able to focus thoughts of heaviness into an area to dissipate tension. Autogenics can also be used to relieve pain caused by poor circulation (by focusing warm thoughts) or by inflammation (by "thinking the area cool"). This is a major step forward in pain control as well as in health enhancement.

BETTER BREATHING

Have you noticed that the way you breathe changes, depending on how you feel? When you feel tense or anxious, for example, you are more likely to take quicker, shallower breaths, using your upper chest. This is actually a part of the stress reaction – the fight-or-flight response (see page 60) – because faster breathing is needed when the body requires extra oxygen for emergency action. Rapid breathing keeps the body on alert, and this is a pattern that can easily become habitual as part of a cycle of strain and tension – particularly where there is a background of chronic pain.

Breathing with the upper chest is inefficient and makes you feel less relaxed and more anxious than diaphragmatic breathing – breathing with the belly. As the discussion of central sensitization (pages 21–4) shows, breathing poorly can increase your perception of pain. When we feel stressed or anxious we breathe faster – and breathing faster makes us feel more anxious. Learning better breathing is likely to help to ease both pain and stressed feelings.

Severe upper-chest breathing is termed hyperventilation, and involves what is known as a paradoxical pattern in which the diaphragm rises on inhalation and falls on exhalation – the precise opposite of what is normal. Upper chest breathing also overuses the main breathing muscles, such as the scalenes that join the upper ribs to the neck. These are then likely to become stressed, tense and painful, and may develop trigger points (see pages 99–100). The main overused muscles, when the breathing pattern is disturbed in this way, are the ones that lie between the shoulders and the neck, and that attach the front and back of the neck to your ribs and shoulder blades. These are the muscles that are most likely to be associated with chronic head and neck pain.

When you fill a glass with water, it fills from the bottom. In the same way, the lungs fill efficiently, with least effort, when you use your diaphragm to fill them from their base. When you breathe into the upper chest, fresh oxygenated air cannot reach the lower lungs. If you inhale when you are relaxed, the diaphragm acts like the piston in a bicycle pump, moving down and drawing air into the lungs, causing the belly to expand. As the diaphragm moves back up to its resting position, it pushes out the air – and your belly flattens. But if you have not fully breathed out, your next inhalation will only involve the upper chest, as you cannot breathe into space that is already occupied by stale air. Upper-chest breathing is therefore shallow and inefficient, and results in more rapid breathing to provide oxygen for the body. The best way to fill your lungs is not to focus on how deeply you can breathe in, but instead to learn how to *breathe out* fully, so that the next inhalation will automatically be deeper.

Breathing is not just about taking in the right amount of oxygen, but also about expelling the right amount of carbon dioxide. The carbon dioxide that you breathe out is derived from carbonic acid circulating in your blood. When you breathe rapidly, in an upper-chest pattern, you may get rid of *too much* carbon dioxide, and

DIAPHRAGMATIC BREATHING
Breathing led by the diaphragm, rather than the upper chest, promotes relaxation and pain relief.

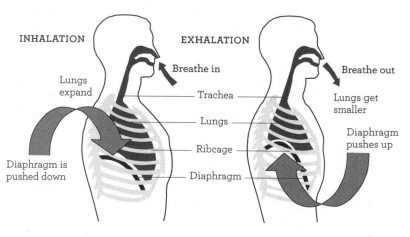

INHALATION

EXHALATION

Breathe in

Breathe out

Lungs
expand

Trachea

Lungs get
smaller

Lungs

Diaphragm
pushes up

Ribcage

Diaphragm is
pushed down

Diaphragm

therefore too much carbonic acid, with the result that your blood becomes more alkaline than is appropriate for your body's needs (known as "respiratory alkalosis"). When this happens certain unwelcome responses take place automatically, in a virtual chain reaction of changes, one of the most notable of which is that you become more sensitive to pain.

Another symptom of alkalosis caused by over-breathing is that your muscles become tenser and more prone to cramp, with feelings of pins-and-needles common. Also, the smooth muscles around your blood vessels become tense, so that less blood (and, therefore, less oxygen) gets through to your muscles and to your brain. This causes fatigue and lack of stamina, as well as symptoms such as difficulty in concentrating together with short-term memory lapses – often known collectively as "brain fog".

In addition, when your blood is excessively alkaline, your sympathetic nervous system is more easily aroused (see page 62), leading to apprehension and anxiety, and even panic attacks. In short, unbalanced breathing means you will generally find that you are more easily upset than normal and, if the nervous system has become sensitized, your pain will feel worse.

All of these symptoms are likely to be worsened when the upper-chest pattern of breathing coincides with a low blood sugar episode, for example if you skip a meal, or during the second phase of the menstrual cycle (due to increased progesterone levels), which may explain some aspects of PMT (premenstrual tension), particularly if cramping and pain are present.

With this in mind, it is not difficult to see why increased pain, sensitivity and anxiety are the almost inevitable results of a breathing-pattern imbalance.

THE SOLUTION: BREATHING WITH THE DIAPHRAGM
Breathing with the diaphragm encourages a calmer mind – indeed, when you breathe this way you create a "virtuous circle" as the

mind and body calm each other down. Some people breathe diaphragmatically without having to think about it, but you may have lost this healthy habit and instead use the upper chest even when sitting quietly (see the hi-lo test, pages 71–73). Being aerobically unfit encourages rapid upper-chest breathing, but of course this is far more likely when chronic pain reduces your ability to exercise regularly.

The simple and safe exercises that are described on pages 70, 72 and 74 should improve your breathing pattern and encourage a calmer mind and less distressed body, helping to reduce your pain. Better breathing – as outlined in these exercises – probably won't feel particularly "natural" at first. But before long, if you practise regularly, your body may remember that this is how you used to breathe, and begin to sense that it is actually *easier*. Once this sinks in, you will find that you start noticing times when stress upsets your breathing, and it will be much easier to switch to better breathing. Regular practice will help get your body used to the feeling and rhythm of better breathing, as well as to the slightly higher levels of carbon dioxide that are retained. You will know you are succeeding in breathing with the diaphragm from the changes for the better in your symptoms, and from your feeling of greater calm, as well as from the results of the breath-holding test (page 71).

A normal, uncontrolled diaphragmatic breathing cycle (in and out) takes about five seconds on average, resulting in 12 breaths per minute, which is 720 per hour and 17,280 per day. If you use the upper chest to breathe most of the time, it is more than likely that you

---

CAUTION: Higher levels of carbon dioxide and an increased supply of oxygen to the brain may make you feel slightly dizzy after or during the exercises on pages 70, 72 and 74. Sit quietly until the feeling passes. It is perfectly normal and will gradually stop happening as your body learns to tolerate the effects of slower breathing.

BREATHING TO RELAX – RELAXING TO BREATHE

Practise this exercise every day for a week or two, before starting on the pursed-lip breathing (see page 72). Do it in a quiet, warm room, at a time when you won't be disturbed, and ideally before a meal or at least two hours afterwards (otherwise you are likely to fall asleep!).

1   Sit, or lie, so you are supported. Close your eyes, relax deeply and scan your body for tension. Start with your toes and slowly work up your legs to your hips, bottom, belly, waist, back, chest, shoulders, arms, hands, then back up the arms to your shoulders, neck and throat, jaw, face, eyes, forehead, scalp. Consciously let any tension go – perhaps by tightening the area and then relaxing, or by focusing on heaviness and warmth (see page 64). Do this for a few minutes so that the body has time to settle.

2   Place one hand on your upper belly below your ribs, and the other on your upper chest (the hi-lo position, see opposite). Without doing anything to modify your breathing, judge which hand moves most, and in what direction, each time you slowly breathe out.

3   Begin silently to count the length of in- and out-breaths, at your own speed. Focus on the out-breath and let the in-breath take care of itself. Ideally, the exhalation should take a little longer than the inhalation, but don't try to control anything, just observe. After each out-breath pause for a count of one – and then inhale slowly and easily.

4   As you relax, you will notice that your chest has less and less work to do. Your chest hand will move less; your belly hand will move more. Without you trying, your breathing will tend to slow down. Enjoy the process for 5–10 minutes.

are a more rapid, shallow breather, and so you will probably take considerably more than 20,000 breaths a day, with the consequences discussed above.

SELF TEST 1: HI-LO

To check for an upper-chest breathing pattern you can use the "hi-lo" test. Stand or sit in front of a mirror with one hand flat on your upper chest, and the other hand flat on your stomach, just below your lowest ribs. Take a medium deep breath and see what your hands do. If the stomach hand moves first and there is not much movement at all of the upper hand, this suggests a diaphragmatic pattern, which is normal. If, however, the upper hand moves first, and/or moves upward toward your chin, this suggests an upper-chest pattern of breathing.

The good news is that such a condition is not a disease, but a pattern of use (like posture) that can be changed by substituting new patterns of use and behaviour. However, like any bad habit, it takes time and persistence to correct.

The exercises on pages 70, 72 and 74 are designed to achieve just that outcome – a new pattern of breathing to reduce anxiety and pain, and to deliver oxygen more efficiently to deprived muscles and brain tissues. By following the exercises for a month or two, you should notice an improvement in your breathing pattern. Use the hi-lo test periodically to see whether your inhalation is starting with movement of your diaphragm. When it is, the hand on your belly will move forward – not upward – at the start of the breath.

SELF-TEST 2: BREATH-HOLDING

Another simple test that you can use to help you monitor how well your body is adapting to higher levels of carbon dioxide, as your breathing pattern steadily improves, is the breath-holding test.

Breathe in normally and exhale, and time with a stopwatch (or a watch with a second hand) how long it is before you feel the need to breathe in again. If it is less than 15 seconds, you are either an

PURSED-LIP BREATHING – ENCOURAGING THE DIAPHRAGM

This exercise encourages the diaphragm to work more efficiently. It can be used to counter feelings of anxiety and reduce pain levels. Perform the full exercise twice a day – upon waking and just before bed. However, if you are feeling particularly anxious, or your pain is severe, you can practise a shortened version for a couple of minutes every hour. This exercise reduces the tendency of the muscles above the shoulders to contract during breathing – which is particularly important for head, neck, shoulder or chest pain.

1   Place one hand on your upper belly below your ribs, and the other on your upper chest. Purse your lips and push the breath out as though blowing at a candle to make it flicker. Blowing a thin stream of air makes your diaphragm work harder, so that its movement feels more obvious. As you exhale your belly should move in, and as your in-breath follows your should belly expand, as the diaphragm draws in your breath. Pause for a count of one after each exhalation.

2   Try to sense the movement of your abdomen – outward as you breathe in, and flattening again as you breathe out. Repeat the in- and out-breaths 10–15 times at your own pace.

3   Once you are comfortable with the rhythm of inhalation, longer exhalation and a pause of one, place your hands on your lap, fingers interlocked, palms facing up. As you inhale through your nose, push the pads of your fingers very lightly against the backs of your hands. This "locks" the shoulder muscles, preventing them from rising as you breathe in.

4   As you exhale through pursed lips, release the pressure in your fingers. Repeat Steps 3–4 at least 10 (and up to 30) times.

upper-chest breather or asthmatic. If it is between 15 and 25 seconds, your breathing is average but still not quite at the ideal level, which is around 30 seconds. Do not try forcefully to hold your breath out, but hold until you have an urge to inhale (a message from the brain that levels of carbon dioxide are building up and that it's time to breathe again).

Your body (and brain) may have become accustomed to low levels of carbon dioxide; as your breathing changes to a slower, diaphragmatic pattern, you will get used to higher levels. As you deliberately breathe more slowly, and levels of carbon dioxide rise, you may feel "air hunger" – a sense of not being able to get enough air. That's why it's good to introduce your slower breathing practice very gradually. By doing this test on a daily basis and recording the result in your pain journal, you will build up a record of your progress and be able to gauge how positive changes in your breathing affect your experience of pain.

"Everything rests in prana (breath)
    as the spokes rest
  In the hub of the wheel..."

The Prashna Upanishad

THE 7–11 STRESS-BUSTER

Rapid breathing caused by stress feeds into a vicious circle of pain, tension and irritability. Fortunately, the opposite is also true – slower, more relaxed breathing helps create a calm mental state and reduces pain perception. Here counting is used to make each out-breath longer than each in-breath, to quiet the fight-or-flight response and boost the body's calming and healing processes. You can do it anywhere, but it's important to have mastered the previous breathing exercises, so that:

- You can sense that your inhalations involve your diaphragm – with movement of the abdomen and not the chest as you breathe in.
- You can sense when your upper chest is involved in your breathing and are able to switch to diaphragmatic breathing.
- You have learned how to slow your breathing down (pursed-lip exhalation and a pause before inhalation).
- And all this is possible without feeling light-headed.

1   Count at your own pace as you breathe, until you find a speed that lets you count from one to 11 on each out-breath.

2   When this feels easy, start counting from one to seven on each in-breath, at the same rate. You will automatically breathe out more softly, so that the out-breath lasts longer.

3   Use counting to help you keep the rhythm going, as you aim to make the out-breath about four counts longer than the in-breath. Counting will help focus your mind, so you are less likely to be distracted by other thoughts. Continue for several minutes. As you practise (once or twice daily), you will identify a comfortable counting speed, so you don't get out of breath. It can be hard to keep count at first, but the technique gets easier the more you do it.

THE POWER OF MEDITATION

It is possible to train our minds to become so absorbed in a task or a thought that it may largely remove awareness of even chronic pain. Studies show that simple meditations – as described in this section – can result in less pain, better concentration, deeper sleep, enhanced mood and well-being and improved quality of life for up to 24 hours after the meditation session itself.

Although many people associate meditation with mysticism and spirituality, one thing that it does not require is acceptance of any particular belief system. You only need the ability to learn to focus your mind or to observe your thoughts as they emerge.

Some forms of meditation are defined as "concentrative practices". These involve anchoring your attention to a single internal or external object, function or sensation. This may be an idea or concept, such as "God is love"; or a word, such as "peace"; or an image – perhaps a candle flame. Another popular concentrative meditation practice involves use of a mantra – a repeated (silently, in your mind) sound or phrase (see page 79). Or aspects of your body, such as breathing, may be used as the focus of your attention.

A different meditation approach is known as "mindfulness". This does not require focused attention – quite the opposite. In the practice of mindfulness, thoughts and sensations are registered and observed as they occur, but they are not focused upon. With mindfulness, an anchor – such as your breathing – might also be used when you become aware that you have lost contact with the observation of your thoughts. Mindfulness is described in more detail in the box, over page.

Whether you use a concentrative or mindfulness method, meditation is one of the most effective means of producing a relaxation response to counteract the effects of the stresses associated with pain and anxiety, and to achieve marked pain relief. During meditation, brainwave patterns alter so that you remain fully awake and alert but deeply relaxed, with your thoughts less likely to dart

INTRODUCTION TO MINDFULNESS

The long-term effects of a regular practice of mindfulness, or other forms of meditation, will be to increase your inner sense of calm – a powerful stress-reducing process that is usually accompanied by reduction in the perception of your pain. Mindfulness asks you to be – as far as possible – in the present, not the past or the future. Practise for 10–20 minutes daily. Over time, you will find that mindfulness can be applied to almost all experiences in your life. Whatever is happening, whatever you are doing, you will be able to observe and embrace the reality of it in the present moment.

1   Sit or lie comfortably, with your eyes closed, and pay attention to your breathing. Without in any way trying to control or alter it, be aware of the sensation of air moving in and out of your body, as you inhale and exhale. Similarly, allow your mind to sense the motion of your abdomen and chest.

2   As you become aware of thoughts, ideas and feelings, whatever they are, observe them without trying to ignore or suppress them. Simply note them.

3   If your thoughts start to wander – no matter how often this happens at first – don't be concerned, but simply go back to observing your breathing. As more thoughts arrive, or awareness of physical feelings or external sounds intrudes, just accept them gently, without judgment or effort. All this time be in the present, where you are, right now.

4   After 10–20 minutes give attention to your breath again, and then to your environment. Sense the room's temperature, your body's position. Open your eyes and observe the space you are in, in the present moment – and then slowly get up and carry on with your life.

about from topic to topic – and even if they do they are simply observed (in mindfulness), without concern.

Regularly applied meditation – of whatever sort – has been shown to lead to a reduction in physical and mental tension, an easing of stress-related symptoms such as high blood pressure, digestive problems, insomnia and feelings of hopelessness, and a definite reduction in perception of pain.

As with so many things in life, different forms of meditation suit different people. As well as the passive approaches outlined above, it is also possible to immerse yourself in a seemingly mundane activity to such an extent that it becomes a focus for meditation. For example, you could meditate – to the extent that you lose track of time – when painting a wall, doing the washing up or even during the simple act of breathing. The only way to find out which method suits you best is to try the various techniques described in the exercises opposite and on pages 79 and 80, and judge which offers you the most benefit in terms of well-being and pain reduction.

Although they may differ in some respects, most meditation methods have certain basic requirements in common. Before embarking upon any meditation program, you should familiarize yourself with the progressive muscular relaxation, autogenic training and breathing exercises described earlier in this book. These will allow you to achieve the best results from meditation if they are already part of your self-care programme, because during meditation you should be relaxed and your breathing regular and calm.

Unless you are employing an active form of meditation, you will need to find a quiet place in which you are unlikely to be distracted or interrupted. It is also important to choose a comfortable, balanced

TOP TIP To feel the benefits of meditation, you should aim to meditate once a day – or twice if you are feeling particularly stressed. Each session should last 10–20 minutes.

posture that you can hold for some time without feeling strain – above all, ensure that you do not slouch. For example, try sitting up straight in a chair with your hands on your lap; or lying on a carpeted floor, perhaps with a soft-cover book under your head to ease neck tension, and your spine flat (put a small cushion under your knees if you have a hollow back).

Although concentrative meditation aims to keep your mind focused on one object, you should not be concerned if you find that your attention wanders. Whenever you become aware that this has happened, you should simply refocus, gently. Visualize the uninvited thought as a pebble dropping into a pond, the ripples gradually getting wider and, as the surface becomes flat and calm again, you can refocus on your meditation object. Indeed, this way of observing intrusive thoughts can be thought of as the start of a mindfulness process: the non-judgmental awareness of thoughts – allowing them to come and go without effort.

" Nowhere can man find a quieter or more untroubled retreat than in his own soul. "

Marcus Aurelius (121–180ce)

REPEAT YOURSELF CALM

Meditating on a mantra – a repeated sound, word or statement – can be an effective way of stilling and relaxing the mind, to reduce the feelings of anxiety that often accompany chronic pain. As with the other methods described in this section, you should practise the following exercise – a form of concentrative meditation – for 10–20 minutes daily to test how effective it is for you.

1   Sit or lie comfortably, with your eyes open. Let your eyes roll upward, as though you are trying to look at your eyebrows, for about 30 seconds, then close your eyes. This mildly uncomfortable stare has a reflex effect, producing the beginning of relaxation.

2   Next, focus your mind onto a word or phrase. You can choose something that relates to your personal beliefs or culture (for example, the Eastern "Om" or "Hare Krishna"; the Islamic "Allah"; the Jewish "Shalom"; or the Christian "Lord, have mercy"). Or the mantra you choose could be a rhythmical word/sound, such as "banana", that holds no particular significance for you. Remember that it is not the mantra itself but the repeating of it that makes it effective in quietening the chatter of the mind.

3   Say the mantra slowly out loud – or silently, in your head – over and over, using it to gently override other thoughts that may enter your awareness. Whatever mantra you choose will gradually become a droning sound in your mind as you repeat it. Imagine that this is the sound of a distant airplane, carrying away all of your unwanted thoughts, and leaving your mind quiet and still.

INSPIRED MEDITATION

The idea of this exercise is to use your breath as a tool to relieve tense, painful areas of your body. Ideally, to test the personal usefulness of the method, you should follow these steps daily for 10–20 minutes.

1   Sit or lie comfortably and, as in the previous exercise, roll your eyes up toward your eyebrows. Hold this gaze for 30 seconds, then close your eyes and focus on your breathing, which should be relaxed and uncontrolled.

2   Silently, in your mind, count one on your first exhalation, two on the second, three on the third and four on the fourth. Then start again. Repeat this cycle throughout the meditation, always counting silently as you exhale.

3   As the exercise progresses, become aware of the rising and falling of your abdomen as you inhale and exhale. If your mind wanders, notice the distraction then, without hurrying, return to the counting and breathing.

4   After about 5 minutes, guide your calming, cooling in-breath to a painful area of your body. Imagine waves of cool air gently blowing away knots of tension in time with your counting and breathing – with your exhalation carrying away the pain. Do this for a few minutes for one area of pain, then steer your breath to the rest of your body, using it to relax tight or painful areas one by one.

5   Complete the exercise by using each breath to bring refreshing energy to the body. After a minute or so of this, open your eyes and slowly resume your normal activities.

THE MIND'S EYE

Visualization is a technique, allied to meditation, in which you create images or scenes in your mind and use them to positive effect – perhaps to bring about feelings of calm, or to ease pain. Visualization is thought to work because your subconscious mind accepts the messages you feed to it, whether they are real or imagined. You can use this power to help you to control and reduce your pain.

For example, you may wish to create images in your mind of a "safe haven", either from your memory or your imagination. This might be a room, or a garden or a riverside – anywhere that makes you feel content, peaceful and secure. It is useful when performing visualization to see yourself in the imagined scene, well, healthy and pain-free. The more vividly you evoke the scene, the more likely it is that you will achieve the desired effect. Therefore, you should try to draw on all your senses, building up layers of sights, sounds, smells and so on. For example, if you are imagining a garden you might first contemplate the sight of a particular flower or tree – the colours of the leaves and the petals, the play of sunshine and shadow, their gentle sway in the breeze – which you also feel as a cooling and calming element in your picture. You might imagine the flowers' aroma, and listen to the sound of bees buzzing or birdsong, as you feel the soft lawn underfoot, touch the flowers or stroke the bark of a tree.

> **TOP TIP** Research suggests that visualization exercises work better if you prepare yourself, just before you begin, with a relaxation technique, such as autogenic training (see page 64), progressive muscular relaxation (see page 63) or breathing exercises (see pages 70, 72 and 74). After a few weeks this preparation won't be necessary anymore and you should be able to incorporate visualization methods as a part of other exercises, or perform them on their own.

WASHING AWAY PAIN

In this exercise you visualize raindrops washing away your pain.
Read the instructions below, slowly, onto a CD or smartphone,
embellishing them with your own ideas. Leave a gap between the
descriptions of different images so that you have the chance to
explore and enjoy them in your mind. When you are ready, play back
the recording. Sit in a balanced posture (see page 78) – remember
not to slouch. (If you choose to lie down, don't fall asleep!)

1   Close your eyes and imagine that you are walking in your
    favourite park. Try to remember it in as much detail as possible.
    Use all your senses, conjuring up smells and sounds as well
    as sights.

2   As you visualize yourself walking, imagine that your pain is rising
    to the surface of your body, transforming itself into pleasant,
    tingling sensations all over your skin. Your pain has migrated
    from deep within to a more superficial level. This is the first step
    in obtaining some relief.

3   It now begins to rain – a few drops at first, becoming a shower.
    You don't mind the rain: it is warm, gentle and refreshing. Enjoy
    these pleasant feelings. After a minute or two, the rain subsides
    and stops. Pay fresh attention to your body, slowly scanning
    it from top to toe. Think about how free it feels – the rain has
    "washed away" the prickling sensation on your skin. Know that
    your pain has definitely eased.

4   You feel relaxed and "light". Stay in your park for as long as you
    like. When you come out of your meditation, open your eyes and
    be happy that you still feel light and free. Carry this feeling of
    lightness with you through the day.

The more elements you can add to the visualized scene, the deeper your relaxation will become, and the more potently you may be able to use other visualizations to have different effects. For example, visualization can be directed specifically toward health problems, as in the "washing away pain" exercise opposite. You might even wish to use surreal images, seeing a painfully inflamed joint as a bonfire which you extinguish in your mind with buckets of icy water; or you could envisage the angry redness of that joint slowly fading to pink as you ease it with cooling breezes. There are no limits to the range of images you can create in this way – the only obstacles are those you might create for yourself.

Once created, visualizations can be recorded onto a CD or smartphone, so that you can return to them easily whenever you feel a need to retreat for a while from pain or anxiety.

As with the meditation exercises, be sure to create a warm, softly lit and comfortable environment for your visualizations. Allow time to perform them in an unhurried way. Sit or lie in a well-supported position, then perform a few slow relaxing breaths, scanning your body for areas of tension and releasing these. Follow any thoughts that seem to intrude, and allow them to fade away as you prepare your mind for the visualization process.

Once you have practised some of the meditation and visualization exercises detailed throughout this section, particularly the visualization of a safe haven described on page 81, you will be ready to apply the visualizing pain exercise (see page 84) to your specific pain issues. The more creatively that you focus on changing the pain, the more benefit should emerge – the only limitation is the degree of freedom you grant yourself.

VISUALIZING YOUR PAIN

This exercise, which uses visualization to engage directly with your pain, should be attempted once you have tried the other meditation and visualization exercises in this chapter. Practise regularly, for 10–15 minutes.

1   Where is your main area of pain? Take your mind to that part of your body. Does the pain have a shape? A size? A colour? Is it cold, warm, hot? And what is the primary sensation that you feel – burning, restricted, sharp or something else?

2   As you ask these questions mentally note the first responses that emerge – so that, for this particular exercise at this particular time, you have a sense of the size, colour, shape and temperature of the pain – and one or two other words that describe its nature. If any thoughts or memories come to you, put these aside to explore later and move on to the next step.

3   Now you can use visualization to begin to change the image of your pain. Start to imagine it as being smaller, less strongly coloured, smoother, more evenly shaped and more tolerable in temperature. Then begin to visualize your pain's primary sensation as changing – if it was tight, release and soften it. If it was sharp, make it more blunt. If it was burning, ease that to a milder sensation, and so on. It may also be helpful to imagine a soft blue, healing light bathing the painful area. Hold in your mind this new image of your pain as being smaller, calmer, softer, more faded, cooler and so on. Perhaps add an image of yourself in a place and circumstances in which you have no pain. After 10–15 minutes open your eyes, feeling alert, positive and comfortable – having engaged directly with your pain.

HEALING SOUNDS

Sound vibrations can have healing properties, and therapists may hold tuning forks that produce vibrations at specific frequencies (for example C) against the body to relieve pain. Sound waves can also be transmitted directly through the skin into problem areas by means of computerized devices. This can help to restore healthy resonance to an area that is out of rhythm with the rest of the body, thereby reducing pain. The processes involved seem to relate to the release in the body of chemicals, such as nitric oxide and endorphins (self-produced pain-relieving hormones).

Research suggests that listening to, or actually playing, appropriate music can induce various beneficial physiological changes. These include slowing your breathing and heart rate, reducing blood pressure and muscle tension, and influencing brainwave patterns in a way that improves your mood and eases stress and anxiety, often reducing pain, possibly because of endorphin release, while also encouraging sounder sleep.

Consult a specialist if you are interested in music or sound therapy, but there is also much you can do at home. Select pieces of music that lift, hearten and relax you, and play them when you feel in need of encouragement, or as a background to your regular relaxation routine. It does not have to be music – sounds such as wind-chimes, birdsong, waves breaking on the shore or the mellifluous voice of someone reading poetry can all have beneficial effects.

For those with a cellphone or access to a computer, there are numerous free or inexpensive apps that can be downloaded to play gentle sounds, such as "white sound", rain and more. Select those that have a calming effect for you and play them in the background as you relax, meditate or practise visualization or breathing.

The use of sound in pain management can also be approached through the concept of the chakras (see page 118). It is thought these so-called energy centres in Traditional Ayurvedic (Indian) medicine

BODY TUNING

The following exercise uses music both to relax you deeply and to rebalance and reintegrate painful areas that may have fallen out of step with the rest of your body.

1   Sit or lie comfortably, ideally in a dimly lit room. Close your eyes. As you listen to a piece of slow music that is at least 10 minutes long, sense your body rhythms by focusing on your breathing rate. Stay with this for several minutes.

2   Then focus on your inner energy system for several minutes, feeling the energy flowing through your cells and organs in time with the music.

3   Now, focus on the music. Feel its rhythms merge with those of your body, so that you become part of the sound. Try to sense any discordant areas of pain and bring them into harmony with the same rhythms. Evidence suggests that joining in with the music, by singing or, even better, by humming, has more benefit than passive listening.

4   Feel yourself to be at one with the music, absorbed by it, travelling with it and possibly joining in with it, until it ends in silence and stillness. Let your body continue to vibrate gently with all its parts now in harmony.

may be influenced by sound. A number of websites (search keywords such as "healing music") offer free-access music for downloading.

We all have different tastes, so it would not be appropriate to suggest specific pieces of music. The important thing is that the music you choose strikes a chord with you. However, quite apart from personal preferences, it has been found that classical music works very well, even for people who claim not to like it.

SLEEPING WITH PAIN

To paraphrase Woody Allen – if you have insomnia, try not to lose any sleep over it.

For sufferers of painful conditions, bedtime can bring apprehension and anxiety. Physical discomfort, and the stressful feelings engendered by it, often leads to insomnia. Indeed, over half of chronic pain sufferers report their sleep being disturbed. This section will show you how sleep works and what happens when it goes wrong, as well as outlining tried-and-tested strategies for improving the quality of your sleep – even if you suffer pain.

Our brainwave patterns change during sleep as we pass through different stages, grouped into approximately 90-minute cycles.

- The first phase within each cycle, called the alpha stage, involves light sleep, also known as REM (Rapid Eye Movement) sleep. This is when we dream.

- The next two phases are known as the beta and gamma stages, in which our sleep becomes steadily deeper.

- Finally, we enter the delta stage, which is the deepest and most restful period of sleep. During this phase, growth hormones, which are instrumental in the repair and healing of the body's tissues, are released by the pituitary gland.

Research shows that tissue-repair functions are most active between ten at night and ten the next morning. Therefore (assuming we don't work the night shift), if sleep is disturbed, repair and recovery are likely to be delayed.

When delta-stage sleep was artificially interrupted in research volunteers, a number of symptoms appeared within a few days,

SLEEP-ENHANCEMENT STRATEGIES

There are many natural ways of improving your sleep pattern without taking prescribed medication. While they may increase overall sleep time, sleeping pills rarely address a deficiency in delta-stage sleep and they can be addictive. Try some of the following instead:

- Ensure that your bedroom is neither too hot nor too cold – research suggests that a temperature of around 62°F (16°C) is generally conducive to sleep.

- Have a small, easily digested protein-rich snack, such as a yogurt or whey protein drink, about an hour before bedtime (but not if you have problems digesting protein).

- Avoid all forms of caffeine (coffee, tea, cola), particularly 3–4 hours before bedtime.

- Avoid active exercise for 3–4 hours before bedtime, as this is stimulating and may delay sleep.

- If you are in the habit of taking a nap in the afternoon, make sure this is no longer than 30–45 minutes.

- Develop a bedtime routine to attune your body to expect sleep, ideally at close to the same time each night. This might include taking a shower or bath (using aromatherapy oils such as lavender), reading, listening to slow-rhythm music or performing breathing and relaxation exercises.

- For the hour before bedtime, reduce lighting levels and turn off the TV.

- If you wake during the night feeling alert, don't toss and turn – get up, go to another room, do a short relaxation routine or read for a short while, then go back to bed.

including tiredness, poor concentration and short-term memory problems – collectively described as "brain fog". When their sleep continued to be affected, the volunteers became withdrawn and felt pain in their muscles and joints. All of these symptoms disappeared when their delta-stage sleep was restored for just two nights.

Nearly half of all sufferers of chronic muscular pain (such as fibromyalgia) experience disrupted delta-stage sleep. They are also likely to have low levels of serotonin, a compound involved in the initiation and maintenance of restorative sleep. When we are in good health, we make serotonin in our intestines from digested proteins. However, if protein digestion is poor, or the synthesis of serotonin is somehow disturbed, the consequences include disturbed sleep, a slowing down of the healing process and heightened pain perception.

In addition to the natural strategies suggested in the box opposite, there are several safe and reliable herbal products and mineral supplements that can often assist in treating sleep problems. These should be taken only on the recommendation of a licensed healthcare provider. For example:

- A protein called 5-HTP (5-hydroxy-L-tryptophan) is said to encourage serotonin production, and is available in health-food stores.

- A combination of herbal products, such as valerian, hops and passiflora – or any one of these individually – can often ease sleep disturbances.

- Calcium and magnesium, taken together at night in a ratio of two parts calcium to one part magnesium, can alleviate muscular tension, and in so doing remove another obstacle to healthy sleep.

- A protein drink, such as one made with whey protein isolate powder, taken 20 minutes before bedtime helps many people to achieve a better night's sleep. If you are sensitive to dairy products, blue-green algae or spirulina powder offer an alternative rich protein source.

NEUTRAL BATH

Another treatment that has been shown to relax the nervous system, and therefore promote better sleep and a reduction in perceived pain, is the "neutral bath" – a bath in which the water is at, or close to, body temperature. Neutral baths are also used to enhance kidney function, or for people who are suffering from anxiety, nervous irritability or insommnia. Note that this treatment is not suitable for people who have skin conditions that react badly to water.

The only special equipment you will need for a neutral bath is a water thermometer. Before going to bed, run a bath as full as possible, with the water temperature close to 97°F (36.1°C) – and certainly no higher. When you get into the bath, the water should cover your shoulders. The effect of immersing yourself in water at this neutral temperature should be profoundly relaxing and sedating. Rest your head on a sponge or a towel. Keep an eye on the thermometer – the water temperature should not drop below 92°F (33.3°C). To adjust the temperature, top up the bath with warm water, but ensure that the temperature does not exceed the 97°F (36.1°C) limit.

The duration of the bath is up to you – anywhere from 30 minutes to two hours is recommended. The longer you spend in the bath, the more relaxing it is likely to be. Afterwards, pat yourself dry quickly and get straight into bed.

YOUR SLEEPING POSITION

The way you lie in bed can have profound influence on how well you sleep, and can directly affect pain – particularly spinal or neck pain, which can severely disturb sleep. Ensure that you have a firm mattress and that your pillows are appropriate for neck support – neither too hard nor too soft.

The commonest sleeping position is lying on the side, with legs and hips aligned (one on top of the other) and flexed. However, because this position leaves the upper leg unsupported, the top knee and thigh have a tendency to slide forward and come to rest on the mattress, twisting the lower spine in the process. To prevent this, it is helpful to place a pillow between the knees and thighs before going to sleep.

If you choose to sleep on your back, a pillow placed under the knees helps to maintain the normal spinal curve of the lower back. A small, rolled towel under the small of the back can provide additional support. Of course, also ensure that your neck is well supported by a pillow.

Some people choose to sleep face down, which can place a great deal of strain on both the neck and back. If this is the only way you can sleep you can reduce the strain by placing a pillow under the pelvis and lower abdomen.

BODYWORK AND REHABILITATION

Many painful conditions can be eased, or completely relieved, by manual therapy. This often combines passive treatment, such as massage, with active rehabilitation exercises that mobilize, stretch, tone or balance dysfunctional muscles or joints. It is important to understand as much as possible about your pain – its causes and prevention and treatment strategies – so that you avoid both "pain behaviour" and recreating problems through misuse of your chosen therapy or exercise discipline.

When you are recovering from pain and injury, or trying to maintain or improve physical function, you should perform exercises in a slow, fluid and measured way, avoiding stiff, jerky movements. The key features are control, concentration, rhythmic precision and repetition, with use of focused breathing to help coordinate movements.

HEALING TOUCH

Rubbing a sore place to ease the pain is the simplest, most instinctive form of touch therapy – massage. This action and other massage strokes (see pages 96–8) can cause a variety of changes that are instrumental in reducing pain and anxiety.

Not only does massage work on a mechanical level to relax tense muscles (and, therefore, ease discomfort), but it also provokes a series of beneficial neural and chemical reactions. For example, by stimulating the nerve endings called mechanoreceptors, massage enables the brain to partially "shut the pain gate" (see box, page 17). In addition, massaging tissues causes them to release painkilling hormones called endorphins and endocannabinoids, while the brain is encouraged to generate its own painkillers – enkephalins – as well as sleep-inducing serotonin. At the same time, massage has been shown to reduce levels of anxiety, while also muffling pain perception. When correctly applied, massage (and other physical therapy methods) also helps to unblock the flow of blood and lymph around the body, reducing pressure in painful swellings and allowing fresh oxygen and nutrient-rich blood into irritated areas.

Studies at the Touch Research Institute, Miami School of Medicine, have demonstrated that as few as two 30-minute massage sessions a week can significantly reduce the pain levels of sufferers of conditions as varied as fibromyalgia, arthritis, pre-menstrual syndrome, multiple sclerosis and migraine headaches.

If you are planning to receive massage from a professional therapist, you should first check that they are properly qualified. Self-massage is also possible (see page 98). Massage is suitable for almost

TOP TIP Next time you feel tense or have a headache, try some of the massage, positional release or stretching methods described throughout this section on the muscles of your neck.

anybody, but do not massage any actively inflamed areas, open wounds or damaged skin.

Massage uses a variety of basic strokes (see page 96) that each have a particular purpose within the context of the treatment, which may be therapeutic or for general wellness (or may merge the two approaches). Therapeutic massage aims to modify the status and function of tissues – to relax them and/or mobilize and decongest them, for example. Wellness massage has as its sole objective the achievement of calm and relaxation – and is, as a result, far more gentle, rhythmical and measured. Massage can be applied locally – for example, to the areas around a particular joint – or it can be applied to the whole body. The basic strokes used in all massage are described on the following page.

An essential qualification for giving a massage is a desire to ease the pain of the recipient, which is why someone close to you, such as a friend or partner, is an ideal candidate for you to massage or for you to receive a massage from. The patient should lie face down on a bed, in a warm, peaceful room, ideally with gentle music playing, and with the area to be massaged uncovered. A light massage lotion or oil can be applied to reduce friction on the skin.

> " Attention to the human body brings healing and regeneration. Through awareness of the body we remember who we really are. "
>
> Jack Kornfield (b. 1945)

BASIC MASSAGE STROKES

Effleurage is a light, gliding stroke, using the palm of the hand. One hand follows the other in a series of rhythmic, caressing actions. The stroke has a calming and relaxing effect, and also reduces fluid congestion by encouraging the flow of both blood and lymph.

Petrissage involves lifting, pressing and rolling muscles in a movement akin to gently wringing out water from a damp towel. As one hand presses in one direction, there is a counter-pressure from the other hand which pulls in the other direction. The idea is to "milk" muscles of waste products and to stimulate circulation. The speed with which this stroke is applied can make it either calming or invigorating.

Kneading is a compressive stroke which squeezes tissues downward and then lifts them, in order to improve fluid exchange and to achieve muscle relaxation in the area. This movement can be compared with the hand actions involved in kneading dough when making bread.

Inhibition is the application of direct pressure to tender areas of tight muscles (or trigger points, see pages 100–101), often using a thumb. Hold the pressure for a minute or more. If this hurts too much, press for five seconds, then ease off for a few seconds. Repeat for a minute to stretch tight muscles and promote better circulation.

Vibration and friction treatments involve small, circular, vibratory movements, applied by the tips of the fingers or thumbs. This has a relaxing effect that can ease chronic pain. Vibratory treatment (harmonic oscillation) can also be achieved with a variety of mechanical devices.

Feathering is a soothing method that is often used to conclude a massage session. It involves a series of light, overlapping strokes with the tips of the fingers, which brush like feathers slowly over the areas that have been treated.

A MASSAGE TO RELIEVE BACKACHE

The following example takes your helper (or you, if you are giving the massage) step by step through a 10–20-minute massage to relieve pain in the muscles of the back. If the person giving the massage has no massage training, it is safest to follow the instructions closely and use basic strokes (see box, opposite) such as effleurage (stroking) and petrissage (wringing).

1 Start by applying massage oil. Begin with long, slow strokes at the lower back. Keep your hands spread out and slowly stroke rhythmically up to the top of the shoulders, applying medium pressure on each side of the spine. Return to the base of the spine and repeat a few times. Keep the strokes firm and rhythmical.

2 Next, target any specific knots and tight muscles you have found. Apply broad pressure to these areas for a few seconds at a time, alternating with circular motions. Don't press too hard. You can also massage down either side of the spine from the shoulders to the lower back, avoiding direct pressure on the shoulder blades or spine.

3 Reach across and push the muscles on the other side of the middle back slightly away from the spine, alternating your hand contact so that as you reach the end of the push with one hand, another push starts lower down or higher up. Each pushing stroke should cover no more than 4–5in (10–12.5cm). Repeat to and fro, so that your hands lightly wring the muscles (petrissage). After a minute change sides and repeat.

4 Continue a combination of these strokes throughout the back massage. Add more oil if your hands no longer glide smoothly over the skin.

5 To finish apply light feathering strokes, for some extra relaxation.

SELF-MASSAGE

Self-massage may involve a mixture of the strokes described on page 96 or only a few repetitions of one of them. Rhythmical application of kneading strokes, for example, can dramatically reduce the pain associated with over-tight muscles or trigger-point activity.

Trust your instincts about where to apply the massage. Try to explore muscles close to where you feel pain, looking for sensitive areas. For instance, if your shoulder aches, search for tight, painful local muscles in the upper arm, or above the shoulder in the tissues between it and the neck, or in the upper chest in front of the shoulder. Often you will be able to identify tight local areas that seem when pressed or squeezed to influence your shoulder pain, and these are the target tissues for self-treatment.

Apply petrissage, inhibition (compression) or effleurage to whatever seems tense, tight and/or painful (but not if it is inflamed – i.e. hot and red) with your fingertips, thumbs or the heel or palm of your hand. Either press directly or apply small kneading strokes, either circular or back and forth.

The intensity (amount of pressure) of the treatment should be as strong as is comfortable to both apply and to receive. On a scale of 1 to 10 – where 1 is painless and 10 is intolerable – you should aim for sensations that are in the 5–6 range. It's best to be gentle at first. You should feel the pressure as a "nice hurt" – a feeling that the pain is being addressed. If you find yourself experiencing increased pain, you need to be far more gentle with the pressure.

If you experience an increase in discomfort in the hours after self-treatment, simply ease up the next time that you apply self-massage. How often you repeat the self-treatment depends on what you feel afterwards – but every second day is usually enough to help, and not sufficient to irritate.

TRIGGER POINTS

Trigger points are localized and extremely irritable and sensitive areas of tension found in muscles. They occur when tissues – usually near the centre of the muscle – become sensitized (see pages 21–3) as a result of local mechanical or chemical stress, or a combination of these.

Trigger points are so called because they are not only painful themselves when pressed or stretched, but – when they are active – they also provoke pain (and other) sensations some distance away from themselves, in "target" tissues. If you recognize these referred pains as something you regularly experience, then the trigger point is actively contributing to your pain. When a trigger point is painful on pressure but does not actively send pain messages to a distant area it is said to be "latent".

Significantly, any stress affecting you as a whole – even something as seemingly unrelated as a sudden emotional event – may irritate the trigger point, making it more active and resulting in pain. The sorts of stress that are particularly likely to give rise to trigger points or aggravate existing ones include: mechanical wear and tear owing to overuse of muscles, injury or poor posture; nutritional deficiencies (especially of vitamin C, vitamin B complex and iron); hormonal imbalances (low thyroid levels, or menopausal or premenstrual situations); dramatic climatic changes and cold draughts; infections involving bacteria, viruses or yeast; allergies; poor oxygenation of tissues; emotional tension; inactivity; and poor breathing habits.

Deactivate trigger points by removing their causes – for example, by improving your posture, breathing habits and diet, and reducing anxiety levels. Pain-reduction therapies that can help range from acupuncture to stretching, positional release and neuromuscular massage techniques (see box, opposite). You can also derive short-term relief of active trigger points by applying an ice pack to the painful area (see page 119).

RELEASING TRIGGER POINTS

If you are suffering pain from an active trigger point, you may be able to deactivate it yourself for a short time, until you are able to deal with the underlying problem. First, you will need to locate the trigger point. Carefully search the muscle that is aching – the trigger will feel like a tight, pea-sized nodular or stringy part of the muscle, probably near the centre, and will be sensitive to finger pressure.

One of the most common locations for trigger points is the neck. To treat a point at the side, or front, of your neck, try to lift and squeeze it between your index finger and thumb, until you feel both the local pain and the target area symptoms (often an aching pain). If the point is on the back of your neck or in the shoulder muscles, press directly into it with a finger or thumb. Hold the pressure for a minute. If this is too uncomfortable, press for five seconds, release for a second or two, then press again – repeat this cycle for up to a minute. Then, stretch the muscle (being sure to cause no more than acceptably moderate discomfort) using muscle energy technique (see pages 104–6) or positional release methods (see opposite and page 102).

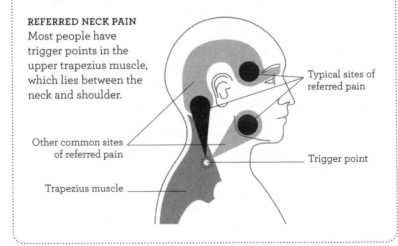

REFERRED NECK PAIN
Most people have trigger points in the upper trapezius muscle, which lies between the neck and shoulder.

Typical sites of referred pain

Other common sites of referred pain

Trigger point

Trapezius muscle

POSITIONAL RELEASE

Derived from osteopathy, Positional Release Technique (PRT or "Strain-Counterstrain") can relieve pain by relaxing tight (shortened) tissues and improving local circulation. Unlike massage and stretching, PRT is safe to apply even to damaged or inflamed tissues.

Many painful conditions result directly or indirectly from tissues (such as muscles, ligaments and tendons) that have been strained, either quickly in a sudden incident, or gradually because of overuse or poor breathing or posture. These strained tissues may stretch beyond their usual length or become shorter than normal, depending on where they are in the body and the type of stress imposed. As a result they are very common sites of trigger point activity.

If you gently ease tissues that have shortened to a position in which you make them even shorter, you can temporarily remove pain from the area. If that position of ease is maintained for a minute or so, the tight, tense muscle (and trigger points housed there) may release and relax – sometimes permanently, but at least for a while. The exercise on page 102) shows how to use PRT on neck muscles, but can be adapted for other areas. For example, if the pain-point (which may or may not be a trigger point) is on the front of the body, bend forward to relieve it; the further it is to one side, the more you should slowly ease toward that side. If the point is on the back of your body, ease slightly backward until the pain reduces a little, then turn away from the side where you feel the pain and fine-tune to release the discomfort. If the point is on a limb, try to shorten the relevant muscles (don't stretch them) by slowly moving them to find the position in which the pain is most reduced. When there are many areas of pain, try starting with those nearest the head and middle of the body.

FINDING A POSITION OF EASE

This experiment uses the sensitive muscles of your neck to show how PRT works. You can tailor it to any area of the body, although you should not apply PRT to more than 5 pain-points in one day, to avoid overloading your adaptive capacity. Your mobility should improve in a matter of minutes, but it may take longer for pain to reduce. You may feel a little stiff or achy the next day, but this will soon pass.

1   Sitting in a chair, search for a place that is sensitive to pressure in the side of your neck, just behind your jaw, directly below your ear lobe. Press just hard enough to hurt a little, and grade this pain as a 10 (where 0 equals no pain).

2   While still pressing, bend your neck forward slowly. Keep deciding what the score is in the sensitive point.

3   As soon as the pain starts to ease, turn your head slowly toward the side where you feel the pain, until the pain drops some more. By fine-tuning your head position, you should get the score close to 0. Stay in this "position of ease" for about half a minute, then – very slowly – bring your head back up straight. The painful area should be less sensitive to pressure. If this really were a painful area, the pain would ease over the next day or so.

TOP TIP To ease discomfort in the chest owing to tight rib muscles, try applying PRT to tender points between the ribs in line with the nipple (for pain in the top four ribs), or between the ribs in line with the front of the armpit (for pain in the lower ribs).

STRETCHING

Stretching is a natural means of restoring suppleness and freedom of movement to areas of your body that have become restricted. It may also relieve the pain that so often comes with muscle tightness, especially if the condition causing the problem is chronic, or very acute (spasm or cramp, for example).

Stretching can be self-applied (active stretching), or it can be applied to you (passive stretching). Whenever possible, you should opt for the former, so that control is vested in the person who can feel the effect of the stretch. Because it is all too easy to overstretch, or to stretch too violently, you should follow these basic guidelines when stretching:

- Above all, stretching should not hurt. If it does, you are performing the stretch wrongly, or too strongly.

- Never use force! If you force your body beyond its "barrier of resistance" (the point beyond which movement becomes uncomfortable), you risk aggravating your condition. It is normal to ache slightly the day after doing stretching exercises, but your overall pain should not have increased.

- You should not stretch inflamed tissues, or areas that have been injured within the previous three weeks or so, as this may interfere with ongoing healing and recovery processes.

Many exercise systems recognize the therapeutic value of stretching. Some use equipment, such as rubberized bands that offer resistance to work against. Other disciplines, such as Pilates, are founded on personalized instruction by a teacher. The following pages look in detail at yoga and muscle energy technique – two methods that are safe, effective and easy to practise without help.

YOGA

The ancient Indian discipline yoga benefits the whole body in a variety of important ways, not all of which are immediately apparent. Most obviously, it helps to relax and lengthen tight or shortened muscles, and to mobilize stiff joints. Regular practice of yoga can also bring about improvements to your posture, thereby averting future musculoskeletal problems. With its emphasis on measured, slow breathing, yoga also harnesses the stress- and pain-reducing effects of a healthy breathing pattern, leading to a calming of the nervous system. All of these positive factors work together to support the body's self-repair mechanisms and, therefore, to promote homeostasis (see pages 30–31).

The practice of yoga involves getting painlessly into specific postures (asanas) – gentle stretches that are designed to relax the muscles progressively without taxing them. The postures look quite different, but they follow a similar pattern. In each case, they stretch a part, or parts, of your body to the barrier of resistance, *but never beyond*. If you find that you are using effort, and are feeling pain, you have gone past the barrier and should stop at once. Normally, you hold a yoga position, without effort, for some minutes, all the while breathing in a slow, relaxed manner. After a minute or two, you will usually have relaxed enough to move further in the direction of the stretch. You then hold this second position – again for a minute or two, by which time your muscles may have relaxed even further, enabling yet another increase in range. The exercise on page 106 shows you how to put these general principles into practice in the Triangle Posture.

MUSCLE ENERGY TECHNIQUE

Like positional release technique (see pages 101–102), muscle energy technique (MET) derives from osteopathic medicine. MET involves identifying a muscle, or group of muscles, that is tense or shortened, and then using a very precise method for releasing any extra "tone" in the muscle to make stretching it easier.

In this method, the muscle contracts without being moved – this is known as an isometric contraction. For example, if you sit at a desk or table and turn your head carefully to one side, you will reach a point where it feels as though it will not turn any further without being forced (unless you are very supple indeed). Turn your head in this way, let's say to the right, and place your left elbow on the desk or table and your left hand flat against your left cheek. Now, using no more than a quarter of your strength, try to turn your head back to the centre, but prevent this movement with your left hand. The force of your attempt to turn and the force of the hand cancel each other out, bringing about an isometric contraction of the muscles that are trying to turn your head. This should not hurt – if it does, stop immediately. After about five seconds release and relax completely. Breathe in and out and, as you exhale, see how much further to the right you can now turn your head without having to force it. This muscle release is known as "post-isometric relaxation". You have just used MET principles on the shortened muscles that were limiting your head movement.

Interestingly, a contraction of precisely the opposite muscle will achieve a similar effect. This time, still sitting at the desk or table, turn your head left until you feel a slight strain. Once again, place your left hand on your left cheek, and try to turn further to the left against the resistance of your hand, using a quarter (or less) of your neck-muscle strength. Again, hold for about five seconds, then relax completely and as you breathe out see that you can now turn your head further to the left without effort. The muscle-release effect of using this method is known as "reciprocal inhibition".

Although these two variations achieve broadly the same effect, there are differences to bear in mind. Post-isometric relaxation has a stronger effect, but reciprocal inhibition is less likely to aggravate sensitive joints. As with any stretching method, you should not apply MET to inflamed or damaged areas.

You can follow the same procedure for any muscle that needs to be stretched, as follows: Find the barrier of resistance. Isometrically

THE TRIANGLE POSTURE

This posture is an effective way of stretching the muscles on the sides of the body – perform it on both sides for a balanced effect. The rhythmic breathing is integral to yoga, and complements the breathing exercises earlier in this book.

1   First, stretch the right side of your body. Stand with your feet a little more than shoulder-width apart, with the left foot turned fully left, and the right foot slightly left. Extend your arms horizontally at the shoulder, palms facing down. Breathing out, bend sideways to the left, so that your left hand can grasp (or touch) your left leg as far down as is comfortable. As you bend, without tilting forward or backward, simultaneously stretch your right hand toward the ceiling.

2   As you exhale turn your head to look at your right thumb. Keep your knees straight and reach your arms as far as is comfortable. You should feel a stretching in tight areas. Relax into the posture, breathing slowly and rhythmically.

3   After a minute, breathe out and, at the same time, ease your left hand further down your left leg, bending a little further to the left. Hold for another minute before slowly coming upright. Repeat Steps 1–3 on your left side.

contract the muscles that are short. After the contraction move more easily to a new barrier of resistance. MET is particularly recommended for relieving pain in muscles that house an active trigger point.

STAYING IN SHAPE

One of the most important aspects of recovery from pain is avoidance of what is known as "deconditioning", which is the precise opposite of being aerobically fit. If you avoid exercise in general, and specific movements (such as stretching) in particular, because they hurt, or because you fear that they might hurt, you can easily fall into a habit of non-use, known as "illness behaviour".

This can lead to a downward spiral where your fear of pain leads to lack of activity, which results in deconditioning of your muscles, greater pain and even greater difficulty in performing normal daily functions. This is a recipe for unhappiness and loss of self-confidence.

Regular exercise is invaluable – indeed essential – in preventing or overcoming the effects of deconditioning, and ensuring that you maintain full body function. Exercise that is appropriate for your particular needs also offers you a way of mastering any fear you may have developed of physical activity, and encourages you to take control of your own pain and well-being. Through exercise you can also cultivate and bolster your levels of motivation and self-discipline.

If you feel unsure about exercising, take heart: yes, pain is a warning to avoid stressing an area, but it seldom represents an absolute demand not to use the part at all, or the rest of your body as normally as possible. Remember the message that hurt does not necessarily mean harm. Clearly, there are exceptions, notably where you have been given medical advice to rest a part of your body (perhaps owing to a broken bone, a torn muscle or recent surgery). Sometimes you may even be advised to rest totally. But what is vital is that you do not make such decisions for yourself, avoiding activity to the extent of causing muscles to atrophy (waste away) – because rebuilding them can take many months of hard work. If you are in doubt, seek medical advice, but whatever you do keep using your body as normally as possible.

SET YOUR PULSE RACING

The beauty of the aerobic principle is that no matter how out of condition you are, exercising regularly can still work for you. If a person has just spent several weeks in bed, a slow walk around the room might raise the pulse rate to an aerobic-conditioning level. A more active person might need a fast jog around the park to achieve the same effect.

You can work out the pulse rate that you should never exceed in your aerobic activity, as well as the pulse rate you should aim for, by feeding your age into the following simple formula:

- To find your maximum pulse rate, deduct your age from the number 220. (Using a 40 year old as an example: 220 – 40 = 180, so 180 is the pulse rate that this person should never exceed when exercising, to avoid straining the cardiovascular system.)

- To find your optimum exercising pulse rate, calculate 3/4 of your maximum pulse rate. (In our example above this is: 180 x 0.75 = 135, so 135 is the pulse rate that this person needs to achieve for 20 minutes three times a week to achieve aerobic fitness.)

As well as helping you to develop a healthy, positive outlook, exercise can improve the functioning of your different body systems. For example, thyroid hormones work better when you exercise aerobically – and poor thyroid function has been linked to certain chronic pain conditions, such as fibromyalgia. And of course regular exercise is vital for maintaining a healthy circulation and cardiovascular function.

To reduce chronic pain symptoms through exercise, research has shown that you should follow a regular program, combining aerobic conditioning, flexibility work (stretching) and, if possible, strength-training activities. The aerobic aspect might include activities such as paced walking, climbing stairs, cycling, swimming or non-impact aerobic classes. Other possibilities include dancing, use of a mini-trampoline or skipping. The key is to tailor your program to your particular aerobic condition (see box, opposite) – with this in mind, you should also check with a qualified healthcare provider before embarking on any exercise regime. In your regular aerobic routine, try not to avoid using any part of the body (for example, through one-sided movements), so that you don't create an imbalance. Above all, whatever exercise you choose should be enjoyable, so that you see it as an integral part of your daily life, not as a tiresome intrusion – otherwise you are unlikely to keep it up.

Stretching and flexibility routines are best followed daily. If you are taking up aerobic exercise, bear the following guidelines in mind:

- To achieve aerobic fitness you need to exercise regularly – at least three times a week, for 20-30 minutes each time. Aerobic exercises are most effective if performed three to four times a week, for 30–45 minutes each time.

- Exercise sufficiently to achieve a pulse rate that guarantees you are exercising aerobically – and this will change over time as you get fitter (see box, opposite).

- Always do warm-up and warm-down stretching before and after aerobic activities, to avoid injury and minimize stiffness.

- Allow two to six months to achieve relative fitness, depending on the length of time since you last exercised regularly, and on your weight in relation to your height. The more deconditioned and overweight you are, the longer it will take, but you should start to feel the benefits long before you achieve true aerobic fitness.

You will know that you are getting aerobically fit when:

- You feel comfortable after exercise and your breathing is controlled.

- Your regular pulse rate (when not exercising) is lower. This will reduce stress on your heart, lower blood pressure and regulate blood-sugar levels.

- Your metabolism improves, making you feel more energetic and probably leading to weight loss (if this is required).

" Walking is the best possible exercise. Habituate yourself to walk very far. "

Thomas Jefferson (1743–1826)

TAKE A BALANCED APPROACH

One reason often given for not exercising by people with impaired balance is fear of falling over. A fall can have serious consequences, especially as we get older. If you suffer from this anxiety, try improving your sense of balance with this simple routine. It will help you train your brain to recognize signals from the tiny sensory receptors in your feet, ankles, knees and pelvic area – proprioceptors – that tell you where you are in space. As this function – known as proprioception – improves, so will your balance. Better balance will benefit you in everyday life – boosting your confidence and making walking and going up and down stairs easier. It will also make the prospect of aerobic activities much less daunting.

1   Stand in a doorway with your arms folded (but ready to use the doorframe for support if needed). Looking straight ahead, lift one foot from the floor and see how long you can maintain this pose without touching the doorframe.

2   If you can hold the pose for 10 seconds, stand on the other leg and repeat the test.

3   If you can't hold the pose for 10 seconds on each leg, repeat this routine several times a day until you can.

4   Once you can balance on each leg for 10 seconds, try practising the same exercise with your eyes closed.

COMPLEMENTARY THERAPIES

Sometimes the rationale behind a given treatment is immediately apparent. If your shoulder were to ache, it would not take much to persuade you to have a massage, for example. In this chapter, however, we will look at some less obvious therapies, such as acupuncture and aromatherapy, which can prove to be just as beneficial when used appropriately.

In evaluating some of the ideas here, try to get a feel for what attracts you and what you will feel comfortable with. You are not necessarily going to embrace all the methods outlined, despite some compelling evidence of their value. Only embark on those that you can accept intellectually – belief in a treatment is vital for its success.

Almost all complementary health professions are now regulated. Make sure your therapist is qualified and belongs to a professional body.

ENERGY AND HARMONY

Ancient Eastern concepts of vital energy form the basis of a wide range of therapies, such as acupuncture (see box, opposite), qigong and reiki. But how do they actually work?

Research into these treatments has demonstrated that they can benefit us in many ways. These include relieving anxiety, pain and chronic headaches, healing wounds, improving blood chemistry and correcting abnormalities in blood pressure.

Significantly, studies have shown that such healing methods can also help enzymes, single-celled organisms, fungi, bacteria and plants to recover from exposure to x-rays or toxins. This proves that – even though the mechanisms are not fully understood – energy therapies exert a real physical influence, that they do not rely simply on the principle of "mind over matter".

A practitioner of, say, reiki can affect a patient's cells, blood and tissues without even touching the patient. This seemingly impossible phenomenon suggests that we need to revise our concept of the physical to take account of the effects of an invisible and intangible form of energy.

Eastern medicine has always incorporated the concepts of balance and imbalance of vital energy into its way of understanding health and disease. Known as *qi* in China, *ki* in Japan and *prana* in India, energy is seen as the feature that organizes all other body systems. It is the basis for therapies, such as acupuncture, that have been practised in the East for up to 5,000 years. Many of these therapies are now widely accepted in Western medicine because of their effectiveness, particularly in pain treatment, but with modern Western explanations replacing the traditional Eastern theories. We should not, however, simply discount the underlying beliefs of a system that has been in place since ancient times, especially now that research in quantum physics has provided insights that, in many ways, corroborate traditional Eastern energy concepts. The results of

ACUPUNCTURE

The ancient Eastern therapy of acupuncture is now widely practised in the West. It involves the (usually quite painless) insertion of very fine, disposable, stainless-steel needles into specific points on the body. Needles may stay inserted for a matter of seconds, or for 20 minutes or more, depending on what the acupuncturist is trying to achieve. Needles may be rotated to produce a sense of heaviness in the area; some acupuncturists achieve a similar effect by passing mild electrical currents through the needles. Other methods of influencing painful tissues include heating the needles – this is known as moxibustion.

Western medicine believes that acupuncture operates by blocking pain messages to the brain (see page 17), as well as inducing the release of pain-relieving hormones. This is in contrast to the traditional Eastern concept of acupuncture as an energy-rebalancing procedure. Regardless of the different theories, research has shown that acupuncture is one of the safest and most effective methods for achieving pain relief – albeit temporarily if causes are not addressed.

this research are already influencing Western medicine – as seen, for example, in the harnessing of biomagnetic fields to jump-start the healing of fractures, and in MRI (Magnetic Resonance Imaging) scans.

The old debate about whether there is such a thing as healing energy or life energy is being replaced by serious study of the interaction between biological energy fields, structures and functions, using instruments that are sensitive enough to detect the biomagnetic fields produced by the body's organs. Minute variations in light and heat emanating from the body can now be measured, and these can be related to different states of health and different stages of healing and tissue repair. Whether you prefer to think in terms of *qi* or of biomagnetism, do not overlook the huge number of therapies that are based on the concept of energy – they may be able to help you. For

CUPPING

In this traditional Chinese/Asian treatment, now being researched for its use in pain management[1], suction or heat creates a vacuum in a glass or ceramic cup that is then applied to the skin. The underlying tissues are drawn into the cup, creating a temporary local congestion with a range of effects, including pain relief. In some cases the cups are left in place for several minutes before being re-applied; or the cup may be moved while the suction of skin is active to cause a pulling of the skin known as gliding cupping. Slight marking or bruising is common after the cups are removed. Cupping is most commonly applied by acupuncturists.

example, practitioners of hands-on treatment methods, including osteopathy, physiotherapy, massage and craniosacral therapy, may unwittingly be using their own energy fields to help to balance those of their patients, thus encouraging the healing process. In contrast, martial arts methods, such as aikido from Japan and qigong from China, train the individual to harness his or her own energy potentials, both for self-defence and overall well-being.

Energy modification is at the heart of systems such as reflexology, polarity therapy and reiki. This is also true of crystal therapy and, to a large extent, of treatments that use light and sound waves to promote health and well-being.

A rebalancing of energy fields may also be what is happening during the "laying on of hands" in spiritual healing. This is widely practised by nurses in North America, where it is known as "therapeutic touch". The therapist's balanced energy rhythms are believed to merge with the unbalanced pulsations of the patient in a process known as "entrainment", to harmonize the patient's energy pattern. The benefits of therapeutic touch have been shown to range from alleviating headache pain to reducing fever and inflammation.

LIGHT AND COLOUR

Seasonal Affective Disorder (SAD), which leads to the "mid-winter blues", is the condition that most clearly tells us just how important it is to have regular, direct exposure to natural daylight. Research has also demonstrated that muscle strength is significantly reduced when daylight, or full-spectrum artificial light, is deficient. In addition, there is evidence that lack of light can lead to increased fatigue, irritability and attention lapses, all of which can be reversed by correcting light exposure. The implications of a lack of full-spectrum light are obvious for anyone who is house- or bed-bound because of illness or pain.

Hormonal imbalances may also arise when we are deprived of light. The pituitary gland, which influences all hormonal functions, has an absolute need for "full-spectrum light". This is only available to the pituitary if light enters the eye without having been filtered through glass. Full-spectrum light differs from the light emitted by most incandescent and fluorescent sources, which almost always lack the blue and ultraviolet end of the spectrum. As mentioned, a major factor in reducing your pituitary gland's access to light is spending too much time behind glass – at home, in office buildings, in the car or wearing wraparound spectacles (or contact lenses). Even being outdoors on a sunny day may not help if you are wearing sunglasses, especially if tinted pink or orange.

To ensure adequate daily exposure to full-spectrum light, you can install light bulbs that are labelled "full spectrum" (these are available from artists' supply stores, if other enquiries fail), or,

> **TOP TIP** During a meditation exercise, try visualizing a particular colour streaming into you, or seeing yourself bathed in that colour. Imagine blue if you feel a need to be calmer; red or yellow if you want to energize yourself.

COLOUR AND LASER THERAPY

In Ayurvedic (Indian) medicine, different energy centres in the body, known as chakras, are said to respond to different parts of the spectrum. For example, the throat chakra, which is believed to have particular influence on the thyroid gland, and to be in need of balancing in cases of insomnia or overactivity, would be treated with blue light. This might call for wearing blue clothing, using blue-coloured light bulbs or drinking water that has been exposed to blue light.

There is no strong evidence for coloured-light therapy affecting physical symptoms directly. However, mood and emotion, which can certainly influence our sense of well-being, do seem to be helped by exposure to different-coloured lights. Canadian and American research has shown that exposure to yellow and red lights produces definite stimulating effects, while blue and black lights are calming.

There has also been a great deal of research and interest in the use of what is known as low-level laser therapy (LLLT) in the treatment of pain, particularly pain resulting from tendon or ligament problems. LLLT requires expert application and is mainly found in physiotherapy or other manual therapy settings. There have been reports of differently coloured lasers offering particular benefits[2]. Lasers are also used by some acupuncturists – particularly for patients who have a dislike of needles – and reports suggest that this approach is equally effective in pain management.

ideally, spend a minimum of an hour each day outdoors. Direct sunlight is not necessary – you get your dose of light even on a cloudy day. If you are unable to get outdoors, and cannot source some full-spectrum light bulbs, sitting at an open window will actually provide the same benefits.

HYDROTHERAPY

Hydrotherapy has been used for centuries for pain relief, and is still a popular rehabilitation treatment in spas and hospitals. Water has remarkable properties, not just in its liquid state, but also in the forms of ice and steam. It has a powerful capacity for transferring heat, whether this involves bringing warmth to a body part or gently cooling it, for example when tissues are irritated or inflamed. When we move in water, our weight is partially supported, so that exercises that might otherwise be impossible can be performed painlessly.

The methods below are safe and effective in modifying pain when used as described. A "neutral" bath is also a recommended treatment for chronic pain, and aches and pains in general (see page 90).

ICE PACK

Because of the heat it absorbs as it turns from solid back to liquid, ice can dramatically reduce inflammation and pain. Ice packs can be used for all sprains and recent injuries, joint swellings, bites, headaches, toothaches and haemorrhoids. Avoid using ice on the abdomen if you have an acute bladder infection, or over the chest if you suffer from asthma, and stop using it immediately if you find that the cold appears to aggravate the pain.

To construct an ice pack, place a 1in (2.5cm) layer of crushed ice onto a towel. Fold the towel over the ice and pin together with safety pins. Lay a cloth made of wool or flannel over the area to be treated and put the ice pack on top, covering it with plastic to hold in the water. (You may need to protect clothing and bedding from the melting ice.) Bandage the whole package in place and leave it for about 20 minutes. Repeat after an hour if it is helpful.

A simpler approach is to use a large plastic bag of frozen peas (suggested as their small size allows the pack to mould to the contours of the area). Wrap the bag of peas in a tea-towel or pillowcase and apply for 10-15 minutes every hour until the swelling and pain reduces.

"WARMING" COMPRESS

This is an ideal self-treatment for: painful joints; mastitis; a sore throat (compress on throat from ear to ear, held by a strap over the head); backache (ideally the compress should cover the abdomen and the back); and a sore, tight chest caused by bronchitis. As the compress slowly warms, the effect is deeply relaxing and pain should diminish. If you find the compress soothing, use it up to four times daily for at least an hour at a time. Ideally, leave it on overnight.

You will need the following: one piece of cotton large enough to cover the area to be treated; one piece of woollen or flannel material large enough to cover the cotton (a scarf is ideal for a throat compress); and some large safety pins to hold it all in place. Wring out the cotton cloth in cold water so it is damp but not dripping. Wrap this around the area allowing the ends to overlap slightly. Next, wrap the outer material around the cotton strip, covering it completely, and secure with safety pins. If the material is not wrapped firmly, the damp cloth underneath will not warm up. It should be more or less airtight, but not so tight as to impede circulation. The damp, cold cloth will soon warm up and be comfortable. Wash the cotton material before reuse.

A note of caution: although comforting, heat tends to cause tissue congestion. If hot water is ever used in treatment – as in the application of a hot-water bottle to a painful area – it should always be followed by a cool application, to decongest and restore normal circulation to the tissues.

CONSTITUTIONAL HYDROTHERAPY (CH)

The alternate application of hot- and cold-soaked wrappings has a non-specific "balancing" effect on the body. Used daily or twice-daily for several weeks, CH can induce relaxation, reduce chronic pain and enhance immune function. The effects of the repetitive use of CH as described in the exercise opposite are cumulative – after a few days there should be an appreciable reduction in general pain, and an improvement in sleep and sense of well-being.

CONSTITUTIONAL HYDROTHERAPY

To apply constitutional hydrotherapy you will need: one double sheet folded in half, or two single sheets; two blankets (wool, if possible); three bath towels; one hand towel (half the size of the bath towels); and hot and cold water. The following instructions are addressed to the person applying the treatment. Before starting, spread the sheets on the treatment bed and check that it will be possible to fold the edges around the patient so that the body is covered from shoulders to legs.

1   The patient should lie undressed, face up between the sheets and under a blanket. Fold back the top sheet and the blanket, then place two folded bath towels that have been soaked in hot water (and partially wrung out) directly onto the patient's body, to cover the trunk from shoulders to hips. ("Hot" means too hot to leave your hand in the water for more than 5 seconds.) Cover the patient again with the sheet and blanket and leave them like this for 5 minutes.

2   Fold back the top sheet and the blanket, then place a hot-soaked hand towel on top of the "old" bath towels and flip all the towels over so that the hand towel is next to the skin. Remove the old towels. Place a cold-soaked towel onto the hot hand towel and flip again, so that the cold towel is on the skin. Remove the hand towel. Re-cover the patient with the sheet and the blanket, and leave for a few minutes until the cold towel warms up. If the patient complains of feeling cold, massage the back, feet or hands.

3   Remove the previously cold, now warm, towel and turn the patient over. Repeat Steps 1 and 2 on the patient's back.

Caution: If you have diabetes, avoid hot applications to the feet or legs, as well as full-body heating treatments. Avoid cold applications if you have Raynaud's disease.

NATURE'S BOUNTY

Aspirin, originally derived from willow bark, is an example of the contribution plants have made to modern medical science. But natural does not always mean safe – arsenic is as natural a herb as you can find. All the same, those herbal medicines that have been well researched, and their safety proven, produce fewer adverse physical reactions than pharmaceutical drugs. The pain-relieving herbs below have been researched for safety and efficacy. Please note, that it is advisable to consult a licensed healthcare professional before taking herbal medicines, especially if you are already taking prescribed medication.

Aloe vera gel has an antiseptic effect when applied to wounds, burns, stings, bites, ulcers and abscesses. The gel can be taken directly from the cut leaves of the plant for external use, or purchased in a preparation to be taken internally to soothe most digestive disturbances.[3]

Arnica has a well-deserved reputation for easing the pain of bruising and contusions, as long as the skin is unbroken.[4]

Bromelain is an enzyme extracted from pineapple stems. It safely reduces inflammation and is useful in arthritis and following trauma. Muscle aches after exercise can be prevented by taking bromelain before rather than after the event. It is important not to take bromelain with food, or the anti-inflammatory benefits may be lost as it helps protein digestion instead.[5]

Cayenne pepper and **red chilli pepper** extracts, rubbed onto the skin, can ease pains following shingles, and those linked to chronic (not acute) joint problems.[6]

Chamomile is known for its anti-inflammatory and anti-spasmodic properties. It can be taken as an infusion, applied on a compress or used to bathe the eyes.[7]

Clove oil is applied directly onto painful dental sites where its anesthetic properties produce rapid relief.[8]

Comfrey (once known as "knitbone") has a long history of use in treating burns, bruises, sprains and fractures.[9]

Cramp bark has strong anti-spasmodic properties, making it ideal for all forms of spasmodic cramp, especially if you have also suffered an emotional upset. The herb can be taken as a decoction or a tincture.[10]

Curcumin, found in the spice turmeric, has been shown to be helpful in easing arthritic pain.[11]

Devil's Claw, from the fruit of a South American plant, is used mainly for treatment of inflammation and arthritic pain.[12]

Ginger relieves digestive pain. Take either as an infusion or in the form of a capsule, available from health stores.[13]

Ginkgo biloba can be taken in capsule form for conditions such as intermittent claudication and other problems involving poor circulation.[14]

Lavender oil mixed with St John's Wort oil can ease general muscle and joint aches and pains when gently massaged into the affected area. [15, 16]

Marigold (calendula) ointment soothes cuts and grazes.[17]

Willow bark (original source of aspirin) as a tincture is used by medical herbalists to ease arthritic pain.[18]

DECOCTIONS, TINCTURES AND INFUSIONS

Herbs are commonly taken in the form of decoctions, tinctures and infusions. These preparations are all simple to create. To make a **decoction** of berries, roots or bark, place the herbs in a saucepan, cover with cold water and bring to the boil. Simmer until the liquid reduces by about a third, before straining into a container for storage in a cool place. A **tincture** is made by soaking the herb in a spirit (typically vodka) for two weeks to extract the active ingredients. The liquid is then sieved through a muslin-lined wine press, and stored in dark-glass bottles. An **infusion** is made in much the same way as tea. Cover the herbs with boiling water and let them infuse for about 10 minutes. Strain into a cup and drink. You may need to add a spoon of honey to make the infusion palatable.

HEALING SCENTS

Safe, requiring no costly equipment and easy to practise in the home, aromatherapy involves the therapeutic use of essential oils that are extracted from plants such as rose, lemon and lavender. Each has specific properties, such as the ability to encourage relaxation, reduce anxiety or alleviate fatigue. Oils can be administered in a variety of ways: they can be added (sparingly) to a bath, massaged into the skin, inhaled directly or diffused in a room. When applied directly to the skin, all oils (except for lavender) must be diluted in a neutral base oil, such as almond or sunflower (follow the manufacturer's instructions).

The role that essential oils can play in pain relief is well documented. Arnica has been shown to ease the pain caused by labour, chemotherapy and surgery. Lemon and lavender oils can help us to cope with stress of any sort, including pain.

Indeed, lavender is one of the safest, most commonly used and most versatile oils for pain relief. To soothe burns and insect bites, it can be applied undiluted to the skin and covered with a dressing. For aches and pains, try adding a few drops to a "warming" compress (see page 120). Other ways of using lavender oil include: tipping a few drops onto a handkerchief or a ball of cotton wool and inhaling from it; pouring 10 drops into your bath; and diffusing it into your room using a steam inhaler or a diffuser. In addition to its direct pain-relieving properties, lavender also increases alpha waves in the brain, which promote relaxation and deeper sleep.

A note of caution: it is important to test for allergic reactions before trying a new oil. Put a drop on the skin on the inside of your elbow and wait 24 hours to see whether you develop a rash. You should never take oils internally or apply them to the eyes, and pregnant women should avoid aromatherapy altogether, unless prescribed it by a licensed healthcare provider. Essential oils should be stored in dark-glass containers, in a cool place that cannot be reached by children. The oils should be discarded when they reach their expiry date.

AROMATHERAPY FOR ANXIETY

The following combinations of essential oils have been used successfully in massages to combat stress and anxiety symptoms. In each case the mixture should be diluted in 1 fl oz (25ml) of base oil. These combinations can also be added to a bath or inhaled using an essential oil burner or simply by adding a few drops to a bowl of hot (not boiling) water. Hold your head over the bowl, drape over a towel and inhale the steam for a minute or so at a time.

- For feelings of tension and anxiety linked to muscular pain and discomfort, blend 10 drops of clary sage with 15 drops of lavender and 5 drops of Roman chamomile.

- For apprehension associated with fear and foreboding, blend 15 drops of bergamot with 5 drops of lavender and 10 drops of geranium.

- For anxiety associated with chronic fatigue, poor concentration and insomnia, blend 10 drops of neroli with 10 drops of rose otto (Bulgarian rose) and 10 drops of bergamot.

EATING
WELL

The expression "you are what you eat" is close to the truth, for the raw materials we take in through food and drink provide the building blocks of that we are made of, and they fuel every process that takes place in the body. Inflammation and tissue healing can be helped by good nutrition, or slowed down by an unbalanced diet. Biochemical disturbances, resulting from food allergies and intolerances, can cause pain or aggravate existing pain.

The information here is for guidance only. Dietary changes are most safely accomplished when you obtain advice specifically related to your condition from a qualified and licensed practitioner. However, one step you can take is to use your pain journal (see pages 36–9) to test the effects of any changes you make. The daily journal gives you a record from which to work, in order to make further changes based on actual information rather than guesswork.

INFLAMMATION AND DIET

To control inflammation through diet, you should increase your intake of fish oils (they contain eicosapentenoic acid, EPA, which calms inflammation); reduce consumption of meat and dairy fats (they contain arachidonic acid, which fuels inflammation); and ensure a high intake of antioxidant foods. Cold-water fish eaten two to three times weekly should provide sufficient EPA, especially if "oil-rich" (for example, salmon, herring, mackerel or sardine). If you do not eat fish, you can obtain EPA capsules from any pharmacy or health-food store. Your body also converts omega-3 fatty acids in flaxseed oil, hempseed oil, pumpkin seeds, walnuts, blue-green algae (spirulina) and green leafy vegetables, such as purslane (also known as Moss rose or Portulaca) into EPA.

DAIRY-FREE ALTERNATIVES

Cutting down on animal fats does not mean you have to give up milk, ice cream and cheese: there are many delicious alternatives that do not derive from animals. Note that many people who have problems with cow's milk cope very well with food made from sheep's or goat's milk.

Instead of animal milks try plant milks, such as rice milk, soy milk, nut milk (almond or cashew), coconut milk or oat milk.
Instead of ice cream try fresh-fruit sorbet, frozen or fresh-fruit smoothies, juice popsicles, fruit ice cubes, frozen rice desserts (made from rice milk), frozen tofu (soy) desserts, fat-free yogurt.
Instead of regular cheese try tofu, fat-free cheese.

To reduce your intake of arachidonic acid, you do not necessarily have to avoid meat altogether. Some game birds and poultry (above all, turkey) eaten without the skin are low in fat. However, duck and goose are fatty – try to avoid.

You can derive anti-inflammatory benefits from a low-fat vegetarian diet that incorporates 2–3oz (60–90g) low-fat cheese or yogurt daily, and eggs from time to time. Research has also shown that a vegan diet (no animal or fish products at all) can have beneficial effects on inflammatory conditions such as rheumatoid arthritis, reducing pain, swelling and stiffness. One study tested the effects on fibromyalgia pain of raw vegetarian or vegan diets comprising mainly vegetables, fruits, berries, seeds and nuts; and avoiding alcohol, caffeine, meat and dairy products. Over a period of three months participants who followed these diets experienced a significant decrease in morning stiffness and pain compared with those following non-vegetarian diets.[1]

Think hard before adopting a vegan diet, and make your decision in consultation with your doctor and a nutritional expert. Vegans run the risk of developing certain nutritional deficiencies, but if you follow a balanced pattern of eating, including – if necessary – supplementation (see page 141), there is no reason why you cannot make a vegan diet work for you. Take special care to include adequate protein by combining different vegetable sources. Eating any two of the following three types of food in the same meal provides the materials to generate protein: grains (such as wheat, barley, oats, rye or rice); pulses from the bean family (such as soy, lentil or chickpea); and seeds (such as sunflower, pumpkin or sesame). Try lentil soup with bread, or tofu (soy) and rice.

Another system that helps dampen inflammation is the macrobiotic diet. This Japanese approach to eating borrows from the Chinese concepts of yin and yang. The idea is to balance "calming" yin foods, such as green vegetables and fruits, with "stimulating" yang foods, such as grains, root vegetables and fish.

Antioxidants that quench the free-radical substances prevalent in inflammation occur in many foods, such as olive oil, blueberries, pomegranates, tomatoes and other red-skinned fruits, green tea and herbs such as oregano, curcumin and thyme. One study showed that 3½ tablespoons (50ml) of olive oil had the same anti-inflammatory effect as 200mg of ibuprofen.[2]

You can also alleviate the pain caused by inflammation by harnessing the enzymes on which your stomach depends to digest food. For example, lipase helps the digestion of fats, while lactase helps you process dairy foods. Proteolytic enzymes enhance protein digestion. Some foods, such as pineapple and papaya, contain high levels of these enzymes, and can be used to tenderize protein-rich foods – for example, by wrapping meat in papaya leaves before cooking. Proteolytic enzymes also have a gentle anti-inflammatory effect – particularly bromelain (derived from the pineapple stem) and papain (from the papaya plant). You can obtain these two enzymes in capsule form from health-food stores. To help reduce inflammation, try taking 2–3 grams of bromelain or papain in separate doses through the day, away from meal times.

" Let food be thy medicine and medicine be thy food. "

Hippocrates (c.460–375BCE)

AN ANTI-INFLAMMATORY DIET

These examples of seasonal meal plans show how you can exclude animal products from your diet and still consume a balanced range of nutrients.

SUMMER

Breakfast Cereal (granola), fruit (particularly blueberries or grapes) and nuts with plant milk (e.g. rice, oat, almond or soy milk)
Mid-morning snack Mixed-vegetable drink
Lunch Cool soup (cucumber or gazpacho) and vegetable salad including tomatoes, beetroot (beet) or (bell) red peppers, dressed with olive oil OR tofu (bean curd) pâté, bean spread or hummus with potato and/or wholegrain bread
Mid-afternoon snack Banana or grapes
Evening meal Wholegrain pasta with tomato sauce and steamed vegetables OR cold potato, grain or bean salad and raw vegetable salad dressed with olive oil
Late-evening snack Fruit sorbet OR frozen soy yogurt

WINTER

Breakfast Oatmeal with plant milk (e.g. rice, oat, almond or soy milk)
Mid-morning snack Warm tomato juice with rye crispbread and tahini
Lunch Warm soup (miso, bean or vegetable) and fresh salad dressed with olive oil and lemon juice OR beans and tofu (bean curd) with wholegrain bread and a raw vegetable salad dressed as above
Mid-afternoon snack Herbal or green tea with dried fruit
Evening meal Thai or Indian-style curry made with vegetables and coconut milk with rice OR Lentil, tomato and vegetable stew with a baked potato
Late-evening snack Rice cake spread with puréed fruit

LEPTIN BALANCING

The hormone leptin helps to regulate appetite, immunity and inflammation. An unbalanced leptin system can result in a "pro-inflammatory state" or Syndrome X[3], which causes an inflated waistline (apple-shaped figure) and increased systemic inflammation.[4] How we eat, sleep and exercise profoundly influence leptin levels and function. To promote leptin balance, and so reduce inflammation, you should:

- Eat a breakfast with significant protein content, such as yogurt or eggs.

- Eat three meals daily, every five to six hours (for example, at 8am, 1pm and 6/7pm).

- Avoid snacks.

- Allow 10–12 hours between your last meal and the first of the next day.

- Finish eating your last meal of the day three hours before going to bed.

- Avoid large meals, and try to eat slowly.

- Reduce your intake of carbohydrates and consider eating more wholesome fat, such as olive oil.

- Try to get adequate exercise – daily if at all possible.

- Do your best to get at least seven hours sleep per night.

- Use stress-coping strategies, such as relaxation and meditation.

OTHER DIETS AND PAIN

The range of health diets can be bewildering – some popular examples that counter specific types of pain, or pain in general, are briefly summarized below. Research has shown that while many people may benefit from such diets, not everybody will. However, some minor modifications – such as increasing your intake of fish or vegetables and reducing animal fats – can only be helpful.

- The **anti-candida** diet is a strict low-sugar, low-yeast regime. It aims to control overgrowth in the body of naturally occurring yeasts such as *candida albicans*. Yeast overgrowth, sometimes as a result of antibiotic use, may trigger allergic reactions and pain in muscles, joints and the digestive tract (and the genital organs if thrush is a feature). The diet seems to be effective, but many people misdiagnose themselves. Seek expert advice to determine whether or not you need to control your body's yeasts before embarking on this type of diet.

- If you are suffering pain as a result of toxicity of any sort, a **detox diet** may help cleanse your system and support liver function. This may involve fasting or consuming only raw food or juices for a period. However, seek expert advice – a detox diet is unsuitable for many groups of people, such as those taking prescription medication or those who are severely underweight.

- The **Hay diet** – said to increase energy levels and reduce pain – is named after its creator, Dr William Hay. A key part of the method involves not eating proteins and carbohydrates in the same meal. There has been no scientific validation of Hay's ideas – any benefit may actually derive from the increased attention that followers of the diet give to what they eat.

- A **low-oxalate diet** may be followed by people who are prone to kidney stones, or painful cystitis symptoms that seem unrelated to infection. Foods rich in oxalic acid (such as leafy green vegetables) are avoided, while low-oxalate foods, such as eggs, poultry, lentils, avocado, cauliflower, nectarines, peas, raisins, bread and breakfast cereals, become a major part of the diet.

- A **Mediterranean-type diet** of fruits, vegetables, grains, fish and olive oil, limiting red meat, has been shown to improve health and ease pain.[5]

"Tell me what you eat, and I will tell you what you are."

Anthelme Brillat-Savarin (1755–1826)

THE EXCLUSION ZONE

Adverse reactions to particular foods and drinks are responsible for a great deal of pain and discomfort. Headaches, constipation or diarrhoea, vomiting, muscle and joint pain, tiredness, skin irritations, palpitations and agitation are just some of the symptoms that these reactions may provoke. Even when they are not the root cause of pain, allergies and intolerances may aggravate existing painful conditions. It can be difficult to identify foods that may be adding to your pain in these ways. In this section we describe the most reliable method of pinpointing any culprits – namely, excluding particular foods and drinks from your diet, then recording in your journal any subsequent changes to your pain levels, especially when they are reintroduced. If your symptoms improve when you are not consuming a food, and reappear when you start eating it again, this is good evidence of an intolerance.

Adverse food reactions seem to be split into two categories – true food allergy (hypersensitivity) and the far less understood phenomenon of food intolerance. Research suggests that food intolerance may result from food toxicity, or it may be that the sufferer is deficient in the enzymes required to digest a particular food – such as lactase, which is necessary for the digestion of dairy foods.

Food reaching the digestive system is usually broken down by enzymes into molecules. Some of these molecules, containing nutrients, are transferred across the lining of the intestines into the bloodstream. Other, larger molecules, containing waste products, are eliminated from the body. However, sometimes the gut wall becomes irritated, which allows the larger, waste molecules to enter the bloodstream. Known as leaky-gut syndrome, this influx of undesirable molecules into the blood can lead to a variety of painful symptoms involving joints and muscles.

Drugs and toxins (such as antibiotics, steroids and alcohol), advancing age, pesticides or additives in food, chronic constipation, emotional stress and major trauma, such as burns, can all contribute to the transfer of waste products into your bloodstream.

Research has identified the foods and drinks that are most likely to aggravate the symptoms of people with chronic muscular pain. These are: wheat and dairy products, sugar, caffeine, artificial sweeteners, alcohol and chocolate.

If you suffer from chronic pain symptoms, you may benefit from conducting a food-exclusion experiment. To be able to draw firm conclusions from such an exercise, you should approach it methodically. Try using the exclusion diet on pages 138–9, or the oligoantigenic diet on page 140, to structure your investigation. Use your pain journal (see pages 36–9) to keep an accurate record of what you eat and the symptom changes that occur.

Bear in mind that when you stop eating a food to which you may be sensitive, and which has been a regular part of your diet, you may experience withdrawal symptoms at first, including flu-like symptoms,

LEAKY GUT SYNDROME
If permeability of the gut wall increases, large molecules may enter the bloodstream, causing pain.

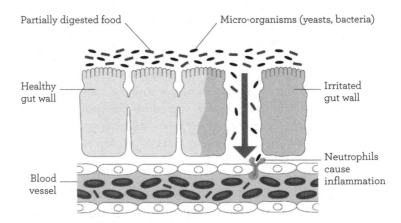

Partially digested food

Micro-organisms (yeasts, bacteria)

Healthy gut wall

Irritated gut wall

Neutrophils cause inflammation

Blood vessel

muscle and joint ache, and anxiety and restlessness. Any side-effects will usually pass after a few days, and can be a strong indication that you may well be allergic to, or intolerant of, whatever it is that you have just cut out of your diet. It can take up to five days for a food you have eaten to stop producing symptoms.

THE NIGHTSHADE FAMILY

Research has confirmed that foods derived from the nightshade family can increase pain levels in some people. The members of this food group include: tomatoes, potatoes (but not sweet potatoes), aubergines (eggplant) and peppers (but not black pepper). Note that tobacco is also a nightshade plant. Vegetables belonging to the nightshade family contain a chemical alkaloid called solanine, which can trigger pain. While there aren't any formal research findings that back the claim about nightshade plants, some people believe they get relief from the symptoms of pain and inflammation by avoiding them.

If you are in pain and wish to test the possibility that nightshade foods are affecting you, leave them out of your diet for two weeks. During this period note your pain scores and symptoms in your journal each day. If you are sensitive to these foods, you should feel the benefit four or five days after excluding them. If after two weeks you feel that your pain has reduced, start to eat the foods again regularly for a week and note whether your pain increases. If so, this confirms that you should exclude nightshade foods from your diet for several months before retesting your reaction to them. If you feel no benefit from the two-week exclusion, then continue to eat these excellent, nutritious foods as normal.

THE EXCLUSION DIET PART ONE: PLANNING

1   List any foods or drinks that you know disagree with you, or that produce allergic reactions (skin blotches, runny nose, palpitations, sudden feelings of tiredness, agitation or other symptoms).

2   List any foods or drinks that you consume at least once a day.

3   List any foods or drinks that you would really miss if they were no longer available.

4   List any foods or drinks for which you sometimes have a definite craving.

5   List the foods or drinks that you use for snacks.

6   List the foods or drinks you have begun to consume more often, or more of, recently (if any).

7   From the following list, highlight in one colour any items that you consume every day, and in another colour highlight any that you consume three or more times a week: bread (and other wheat products); milk; potatoes; tomatoes; fish; cane sugar or its products; breakfast cereals; sausages or preserved meat; cheese; coffee; rice; pork; peanuts; corn or its products; margarine; beetroot or beet sugar; tea; yogurt; soy products; beef; chicken; alcohol; cake; biscuits (cookies); citrus fruits; eggs; chocolate; lamb; artificial sweetener; soft drinks; pasta.

THE EXCLUSION DIET PART TWO: ACTION

1   Exclude from your diet the item you have listed and highlighted most often in Part One. If there is a tie for first place, it doesn't matter which you choose to exclude first – toss a coin if you like. For most people the foods that provoke pain will appear both as answers to the questions and also in the highlighted list. The foods most likely to offend are dairy products, grains (especially wheat), soy products, nightshade vegetables (see page 137) and citrus fruits.

2   If after a week your symptoms (muscle or joint pain, fatigue and so on) have improved, you should maintain the exclusion for two or three weeks more, before reintroducing the excluded food or drink to see whether the symptoms return. If they do (commonly after the second or third time you consume the reintroduced food), you will have confirmed that your body is better off, for the time being at least, without the food you have identified.

3   Repeat the exclusion process for the next-most frequently listed item on your questionnaire. Work down your list, always selecting the next-most frequently mentioned item. If you find a particular food causes symptoms, allow a week before starting to test the next food on the list.

4   Remove from your diet any items that tested "positive" in your exclusion experiment. Wait at least six months before retesting the problem foods or drinks. By then you may have become desensitized to them and be able to tolerate them again – if not all the time, then once every four to five days.

THE OLIGOANTIGENIC DIET

Another way to identify foods to which you are sensitive is to try a modified oligoantigenic exclusion diet, which has been shown to be very effective in relieving many pain-related conditions, including migraine.[6] Exclude at the same time for three to four weeks all the foods and drinks listed below as "forbidden". If you feel less pain after this period, reintroduce items that you had previously eaten, one at a time, leaving four to five days between each reintroduction. If, when you reintroduce a particular food, your pain symptoms recur, eliminate that food from your diet for at least six months. Allow five days for your body to clear all traces of the offending food before continuing the gradual reintroduction of the remaining excluded items.

Fish: white fish, oily fish allowed; smoked fish forbidden.
Vegetables, pulses: none is forbidden, but people with bowel problems should avoid beans, lentils, Brussels sprouts and cabbage.
Fruits: all are forbidden, except banana, passion fruit, peeled pear, pomegranate, papaya (paw-paw) and mango.
Cereals: rice, sago, millet, buckwheat and quinoa are allowed; wheat, oats, rye, barley and corn are forbidden.
Oils: sunflower, safflower, linseed and olive are allowed; corn, soy, "vegetable" and nut (especially peanut) are forbidden.
Dairy: all dairy is forbidden – including cow's milk and all its products including all goat-, sheep- and soy-milk products.
Drinks: herbal teas are allowed; tea, coffee, fruit squashes, citrus drinks, apple juice, alcohol, tap water and carbonated drinks are forbidden.
Miscellaneous: sea salt is allowed; all yeast products, chocolate, preservatives, food additives, herbs, spices, honey, eggs, margarines and sugar of any sort are forbidden.

SUPPLEMENTS

We have already seen that boosting your intake of EPA (found in fish oil and some plants) and certain enzymes can ease pain, because of their natural anti-inflammatory properties (see pages 128–9). There is also strong evidence in favour of supplementing other nutrients to help ease pain – ranging from calcium and magnesium to various B-vitamins, and essential fatty acids found in evening primrose oil.

However, you will only benefit from taking a supplement if you are deficient in the nutrient in question in the first place. As a result, it is not always advisable to self-prescribe nutrient supplements. For a start, supplements can be expensive, and buying those you do not need can be unnecessarily costly.

Secondly, certain vitamins and minerals, such as selenium and vitamin B6, can cause toxic reactions if you exceed the recommended dose. To get the most out of supplements, you should consult a licensed nutritional expert, such as a dietician, nutrition counsellor or naturopath. By seeking expert advice you will avoid falling into the trap of unnecessary, and potentially unbalanced, supplementation.

Having said that, there is certainly no harm in taking a well-formulated multivitamin or multimineral supplement to ensure that at least the basic requirements of the body are being met. And calcium and magnesium will aid muscle and bone health, particularly if taken pre- and post-menopausally by women to protect against osteoporosis in later years.

TYPES
OF PAIN

There are pains that can be described as a "nice hurt" (as in deep massage, for example, when the therapist's hands touch what seems to be the source of discomfort in a satisfying way), and some that are a background nuisance, or are so familiar and non-threatening that they can almost be ignored. Then there are the pains that are awful, that dominate all thinking and prevent normal functioning. And then there are pains that lie somewhere in between.

Benjamin Franklin said that the only two certainties in life were death and taxes, but he could have added pain to his uncomfortable list, because none of us escapes it. This chapter presents examples of types of pain, from the everyday to the severe, and offers specific advice on how to ease them. The hope is that increased understanding of the choices available to us will help us to handle pain as effectively as possible.

READING THE SIGNS

One way of looking at pain is as the body's means of communicating distress. Pain speaks in many different ways – it may shriek at you, or nag or grumble. By heeding the tone and nuances of this language, you can gain important insights into the nature of your condition, and plan your recovery accordingly.

Some pains are clearly local, and have little bearing on your general health. Strains, sprains, burns, bruises, joint injuries and localized osteoarthritic changes, resulting from overuse or injury, can all be treated for what they are – local conditions. Acute local conditions will usually recover in a matter of days or weeks, if not aggravated during the recovery phases of the natural healing process. Long-standing, chronic local problems – such as arthritis of a wrist or a knee – need to be evaluated to see how you can modify everyday patterns of use to reduce stress on the joint. You should also consider whether these problems can be helped by strategies such as hydrotherapy, acupuncture, exercise, direct manual treatment, medication or changes to your diet.

Other pains may derive from conditions that affect the body as a whole. In these cases, you will invariably need to adopt a broad approach, considering nutritional, emotional, hormonal, circulatory and other bodywide influences. Generalized pain-producing problems include rheumatoid arthritis and fibromyalgia, which require treatment of the whole person – mind and body – as well as treatment to ease local symptoms (see Sensitization, pages 21–24).

Other pains can combine local and general elements, such as sciatic pain in the leg derived from a back condition; or trigger-point pain that is felt in one place, but comes from a trigger in a distant muscle; or a headache originating from neck strain. You need to work in conjunction with a healthcare professional to address the root cause of such pain. To deal with such things locally is a temporary solution at best.

MAKING SENSE OF YOUR PAIN

The following questions will help you to analyze your pain in a methodical way, either to prepare yourself for a consultation or to devise your own self-help strategies.

- What has caused my pain?

- Is the pain constant or does it come and go?

- If it is not constant, are there any activities that seem to bring it on?

- Is it local, or part of a general condition or a combination of the two?

- Has it been referred to the area that hurts by another part of my body?

- Is it acute, chronic or an acute flare-up of an old (chronic) problem?

- If the pain is acute, is the painful area inflamed?

- What eases the pain? What aggravates it?

- What can I do to aid the healing process? What should I avoid doing?

- How can I best engage my inner resources to deal with my pain, and to overcome the restrictions it imposes on me?

As well as working out whether a pain is local, general or referred, you should assess whether it is acute or chronic. Treatment strategies will vary depending on the answers you give to the questions in the box above. If your condition is acute, do not apply any treatment that might increase inflammation or other acute symptoms, or interfere with the tissue healing. Chronic problems require a different approach. For example, to ease pain caused by joints or muscles that have tightened over time, you might try regular focused stretching and strengthening methods. A word here about inflammation. This is a key aspect of the healing process. If it is causing pain, you might choose to reduce it to more comfortable levels through natural strategies, such as hydrotherapy or dietary changes, rather than by taking medication.

As we have seen, there are many strategies that can offer a measure of relief from painful conditions, including relaxation and visualization methods, better nutrition and aerobic activity. All of these reduce stress levels, improve circulation and make the body's defence-and-repair systems operate more efficiently. And there are also the numerous specific and local methods, discussed elsewhere in this book, that can help as first aid, or provide short-term relief.

The built-in ability of the body to recover from illness and impaired function – homeostasis – is the greatest health-guarantor we have. This is the "physician within", working tirelessly toward recovery, which we can assist by removing obstacles to health, and which we need to harness when we begin to feel despair. Three key features examined in the first two chapters of this book are essential for the tackling of any pain – we need to understand the pain process, achieve some control over it and exert the powerful command of mind over body.

COMMON PAINS

Thankfully, most people's experience of pain is restricted to minor bumps, bruises, stings, cuts and burns. Listed here are some of the most common causes of "minor" pain, together with first-aid measures that may prove to be helpful.

To treat **bruises**, dissolve one or two arnica triple-strength homeopathic pillules (available from many pharmacies or health-food stores) under your tongue every 30 minutes until discomfort starts to ease.

When tackling a **burn or scald**, first remove the source of the burn and any clothing or jewelry in the area of the injury. If the burn was caused electrically, seek emergency assistance. If the area involved is less than 1in (2.5cm) across, treat it yourself. If larger, get expert help. Place the burn under cold running water immediately and keep it there for no less than 10 minutes, longer if possible, or until medical help arrives. Never use butter, oil or grease on a fresh burn and do not break any blister. Cover with cling film or a light gauze bandage until you receive expert advice. Use a diluted lavender-oil dressing once healing is underway.

To relieve **muscle cramp**, either stretch the muscle immediately or find the centre of the cramp and apply strong thumb pressure until it eases. Check your nutritional balance, particularly of sodium, calcium and magnesium, with a qualified practitioner.

To get to the root cause of a **mouth ulcer**, you will probably need to seek medical advice. However, first aid may be helpful: place a moistened tea bag over the ulcer for as long as possible; or suck an ice cube, trying to keep it over the ulcer site.

Steam inhalation is a useful first aid for easing painful **sinus inflammation**. Pour boiling water into a bowl and add a drop of pine or eucalyptus oil. Place your face over the bowl, with a towel draped over your head, for 10–15 minutes. Repeat this treatment several times a day. Pain resulting from sinus congestion can also be eased by humming strongly (try to get the vibration to focus on the painful area) as this releases nitric oxide from the tissues of the nose, which helps the process of decongestion.

Insect stings are most commonly inflicted by bees and wasps. If stung by a bee, remove the sting using tweezers (with wasp stings there is nothing to remove). Place the area under cold running water for at least 10 minutes and then apply vinegar or lemon juice, or a paste made from bicarbonate of soda, to neutralize the venom. If there is any sign of an allergic reaction – say, difficulty breathing or swallowing – seek medical attention urgently.

"Pain is inevitable. Suffering is optional."

Buddhist proverb

A PAIN-BY-PAIN DIRECTORY

On the following pages we take a tour of the body's major trouble spots, in each case looking at how pain most commonly arises there and suggesting appropriate therapies and strategies described more fully in earlier chapters.

HEADACHES

Headaches are common, and usually not life-threatening. However, it is wise to get medical advice if a headache is out of the ordinary (for example, accompanied by visual disturbances, high temperature, very stiff neck or throbbing; or if the pain comes on after a sudden head movement or blow to the head). There are three main types of headache.

- A **tension headache** is characterized by aching (seldom throbbing) and a feeling of tightness in the temples (or the top or back of the head), as well as discomfort in the neck and/or shoulders.
- The classic **migraine** is usually one-sided, with severe pain (throbbing, pounding or piercing) lasting for many hours or days. Migraines may be heralded by an aura of flashing lights, or by nausea or extreme sensitivity to light. Their cause remains unclear – they may be triggered by weather changes, or bright or flickering lights, or stressful episodes or particular foods. If attacks coincide with menstruation, hormonal irregularities may be the cause.
- Like migraines, **cluster headaches** are usually one-sided, but, unlike most migraines, they start without warning. Typically lasting about an hour, they involve severe pain in the eye, temple, face and neck, and sometimes the teeth and shoulders. Cluster headaches are more common in men and are often accompanied by sweating and a running nose or eyes, suggesting a food intolerance or allergy background.

Some treatments are appropriate for all three types of headache. These include relaxation and visualization methods, especially autogenic training and biofeedback – but they only work for migraines if you apply them at the first sign of the headache. Certain aromatherapy oils – particularly lavender and chamomile – can assist the relaxation process, as can soothing herbal teas, such as chamomile, rosemary, lavender and ginger. Acupressure and acupuncture can also be effective, although for migraines you will usually need to follow a full course of acupuncture rather than expecting a single treatment to work.

Certain therapies work particularly well for tension headaches. For example, many tension headaches derive from trigger-point activity, and so may benefit from manual treatment of the muscles housing the triggers. Hydrotherapy can often help – particularly the alternating of hot and cold applications to the back of the neck, or a "warming" compress to the forehead or back of the neck combined with a hot foot bath. At the simplest level, you should keep warm and rest, eat only light foods and avoid alcohol.

Rest is also important for migraines, but keep cool rather than warm. Other strategies include massage and manipulation – especially of the upper-neck area – using osteopathic, chiropractic or craniosacral methods. Studies have shown that these techniques can prevent migraines (in some cases permanently), and may also help to abort attacks that are already underway. Pressing on trigger points on the temple, base of the skull or lower neck may be effective, especially if the pressure initially increases or reproduces your symptoms.

> **TOP TIP** Over-the-counter painkillers and prescribed migraine drugs can help to ease headaches. However, most carry the risk of side-effects, such as nausea and drowsiness. Regular use of such medication also seems to increase the frequency of attacks.

HOW TO AVERT A TENSION HEADACHE

If applied before the headache is well established, this method can ward off tension headaches, but not migraines or cluster headaches.

- Place 2 gallons (9 litres) of hot water (not scalding) into a bowl large enough to accommodate both feet. Stir 1 to 2 teaspoons of mustard powder into the bowl and immerse your feet, up to the ankles.

- Wrap a large bag of frozen peas in a towel and place this behind your neck. (If you sit on an upright chair against a wall, you can lean back onto the towel containing the peas.)

- Spend at least 10 minutes in this position and then lie down and rest.

Herbal feverfew tablets (or eating one feverfew leaf daily) reduce the frequency and intensity of migraines for some people, but are of no help once a migraine has started. Studies have shown the herb butterbur to offer relief from migraine headaches, and to prevent recurrence in many cases. Migraines were shown to have been prevented in over 60 percent of chronic sufferers who used the nutritional supplement CoEnzyme Q10 (CoQ10).[1]

Advocates of homeopathy claim good results with migraines – but you should seek expert advice, rather than embarking on a course of self-prescribed treatment.

Certain foods appear to provoke migraines, so record in your pain journal everything you ate in the 12 hours before an attack. Key suspects include: coffee (or other caffeine drinks); alcohol; tyramine-rich foods (such as mature cheese, chocolate and some nuts); nitrite-rich foods (including most cured or preserved meats); foods rich in monosodium glutamate (MSG); and artificial sweeteners. An oligoantigenic diet may help you to identify the culprits.

Low-blood sugar episodes (hypoglycemia) seem to provoke migraines in some people, suggesting that you should not skip meals, and that you should follow a balanced diet that excludes high-sugar items. Deficiencies in specific minerals and vitamins may also be a factor. However, you should consult a qualified nutritionist rather than prescribing supplements for yourself.

JAW, FACE AND TOOTH PAIN

Pain in, or deriving from, the jaw (temporomandibular joint, or TMJ) can be severe. TMJ syndrome may involve difficulty in opening the mouth fully and in chewing, as well as noisy cracking and grating in the joint. There may also be active trigger points in the jaw muscles, which can be treated manually using neuromuscular massage, pain-killing injections or acupuncture.

The causes of TMJ pain can include dental imbalances (malocclusion), which can be corrected by certain dental practitioners, especially those who offer craniosacral therapy. Postural habits that stress the neck and head – for example, sitting with rounded shoulders and your head forward – may also be to blame. If this is the case, you should consult a chiropractor, specialist osteopath, physiotherapist or an expert in postural retraining, such as an Alexander Technique or Pilates teacher. Excessive use of chewing gum, as well as habitual tooth grinding (bruxism), which is often linked with anxiety, are other potential factors. Bruxism can be countered by wearing a plastic mouthguard, especially at night. Relaxation, autogenic training and visualization practices will help to ease the psychological stress that can be the root cause of many TMJ problems.

Pressing the acupuncture points in the webbing between the thumb and index finger of each hand, closer to the finger than the thumb, can relieve toothache, headache and TMJ pain. Press firmly

A TRIATHLON FOR YOUR JAW

This three-stage routine for alleviating TMJ pain is easy to carry out yourself – try it three times a day. Although the effects vary from person to person, you could expect to notice a reduction in your jaw pain after about a week.

1   Sit with one elbow on a table, and your clenched fist supporting your jaw. Rest (don't press) the tip of your tongue against the middle of your lower front teeth – this ensures your jaw opens and closes symmetrically. Try to open your mouth against the resistance of your fist, which should slow the opening but not stop it altogether. Open and close your mouth five times, slowly, against resistance; and then open and close it five more times, slowly, without the hand resistance. Make sure the lower teeth stay behind the upper teeth on closing, with the tongue held as described above throughout.

2   Relax, then slowly open your mouth as far as you can without pain to stretch the muscles controlling the jaw. Hold for 5–10 seconds. Repeat this stretch once more.

3   Sitting up straight, place the tip of your tongue as far back on the top of your mouth as you can. While the tongue is in this position, slowly and gently open and close your mouth a few times as widely as you can without causing pain. This activates particular muscles (the retrusive group) and helps to reduce tension in them.

TOP TIP Try these first aids for toothache: wash your mouth frequently with half a teaspoon of salt (or five drops of myrrh tincture) dissolved in a glass of warm water; or apply clove oil or brandy to the painful area using a cotton-tipped applicator. TENS and acupuncture can also help in the short term.

with your other thumb for up to a minute at a time. (Do not press areas of inflammation, broken skin or varicose veins.)

NECK AND SHOULDER PAIN

Unless you have suffered a specific injury (see below), pain in the neck and shoulders usually comes from a habitual posture that puts stress on the muscles in this area. The most common culprit is a round-shouldered, head-forward posture, which not only strains the muscles supporting and moving the neck, but also crowds the upper chest, causing breathing imbalances. As muscles gradually become excessively tense they also develop trigger points, which can refer pain into distant tissues. Avoid seated and lying postures that aggravate the problem by choosing appropriately designed furniture, and by using pillows to support the neck in a non-stressful sleeping position. Treatment should aim to stretch the tightened muscles, deactivate trigger points, tone up weakened muscles and improve posture (see opposite). Physiotherapists, chiropractors, specialist osteopaths and neuromuscular massage therapists can all help.

Another source of neck and shoulder pain is "whiplash" injury, often caused by a car accident. Usually these injuries heal within a few months, but damage to delicate nerve structures, disks and joints may lead to long-term pain and restricted mobility. In a few cases, small muscles at the base of the skull are so severely affected that they atrophy, giving rise to fibromyalgia. Consult an expert if you have a whiplash injury that is still uncomfortable. Methods that may aid your recovery include: acupuncture and TENS;

> **TOP TIP** Many kinds of neck pain, including whiplash injuries, may involve activated trigger points. Try using positional release technique (see pages 101–102) to treat these trigger points.

REBALANCE YOUR POSTURE

Many of us spend long periods of our working day at a desk, hunched over paperwork or a computer keyboard. These, among other activities, can lead to an unbalanced, round-shouldered posture that pushes your head forward. The following exercise should help to ease the muscles in the neck and shoulders that are stressed as a result of such a posture. Do it hourly during the time you spend working at a desk.

1 Perch on the edge of a chair or stool, with your feet flat on the floor, slightly wider apart than your hips, toes pointing slightly outward.

2 Tucking your chin in slightly, allow your arms to hang straight down with your palms facing forward.

3 As you breathe in, turn your arms so that your thumbs face backward, and stretch out your fingers. At the same time, lift your breast bone slightly forward and up, and very slightly arch the lower back. As you slowly breathe out, relax and let your hands return to the starting position. Repeat five times.

anti-inflammatory nutritional and hydrotherapy measures; manual and exercise (such as Pilates) therapy; and self-applied relaxation and visualization exercises.

Upper-chest breathers automatically overuse and stress the scalene muscles between the shoulders and the neck. Trigger points are likely to develop here, referring pain to the neck and head. Learning slow, diaphragmatic breathing will relieve these overworked muscles (see pages 66–74).

ARM AND HAND PAIN

The arms and hands are particularly susceptible to repetitive strain injuries, which include tenosynovitis ("tennis elbow") and carpal tunnel syndrome (affecting the hand and wrist).

"TENNIS ELBOW" RELIEF

This exercise uses muscle energy technique (see pages 104–106) to relieve the inner elbow pain of "tennis elbow". (This can be caused by any activity that leads to overuse of the elbow joint – not just playing tennis.) If you do the exercise no more than once a day, you should feel benefit after about a week.

1   Sitting with your painful elbow on a table, forearm upright, palm facing forward, gently bend your wrist back with your other hand, so that your fingers point toward your face. Bend only as far as you can without it hurting. With your wrist in this bent position, use your other hand to resist an attempt to bring the wrist back to its neutral position. Maintain this light isometric contraction of the flexor muscles in your forearm for 7–10 seconds.

2   Relax, and then press lightly on the palm of the hand being treated to bend it back further than was possible in Step 1. Stretch the flexor muscles in this way for at least 20 seconds.

3   Repeat Steps 1 and 2 at least once more.

4   Then to stretch the back of your forearm, place your elbow on the table, forearm upright, palm toward your face. Bend your wrist back as before and repeat the method described above.

If you work at a desk, you can take steps to minimize your chances of developing such conditions:

- Avoid typing for more than four hours a day.
- Stretch gently (without producing pain) for three minutes every half hour.
- Pay attention to your posture, the height of your desk and the position of equipment such as your computer.
- Undertake general, regular exercise.
- Monitor your stress levels.

If you do develop an "overuse" problem, it can be treated with rest (and sometimes splinting of the wrist), physiotherapy or even surgery (for example, to release trapped nerves). If the area is inflamed, reduce swelling through diet and hydrotherapy (especially an ice pack). Any trigger points giving rise to the pain should be deactivated, for example using neuromuscular massage or acupuncture.

If the condition is severe, cortisone injections may be an appropriate option. However, repeated application can weaken tissues. Before resorting to cortisone, you should try conservative methods, such as ergonomic and postural re-education, TENS, acupuncture and bodywork – under expert supervision.

BACKACHE

No pain provokes more visits to the doctor than backache, although – even without treatment – it usually gets better within a few weeks. However, if pain persists for more than two to three weeks you must seek professional advice, as the list of potential causes is so varied. This can include disk problems; trapped nerves; irritated, restricted or inflamed joints; muscular irritation or spasm; or trigger-point activity. Occasionally, persistent back pain can be caused by other internal problems, such as kidney disease or a gall-bladder condition.

Advice for backache will depend on its cause. However, there are some general principles. Above all, do not do anything that aggravates the pain. It is important to work out the difference between "hurt" and "harm". Gentle back stretches (see opposite) may hurt a little, but as long as they do not aggravate your existing back pain, they are unlikely to be doing harm – and may well help.

Avoid complete rest or using a back rest for more than a few hours at a time, unless this is advised by an expert or pain is extremely acute. Unused muscles rapidly lose mass and strength, which will slow down your recovery. Rehabilitation from chronic back pain almost always demands the strengthening of spinal and abdominal stabilizing muscles, requiring advice and instruction from an expert, such as a specialist osteopath, a physiotherapist or a chiropractor, ideally working in collaboration with a Pilates instructor.

There are various measures for all kinds of back pain, such as deactivation of trigger points – consult a neuromuscular or massage therapist. A licensed massage therapist can help alleviate your back pain, particularly by targeting specific trigger points. Acupuncture and TENS can also ease chronic back pain, if only temporarily.

If your pain features tight muscles either side of your spine, try lying on two tennis balls in a sock (tied off to stop them escaping), so that one is on each side of your spine. By slowly moving around on the balls, you can get pressure right into the tight, sore spots that need to relax. Use this technique as often as you feel it helpful, always following up with a gentle stretch for the painful area.

> **TOP TIP** Looked at in profile, the spine is curved in an "S" shape. When you stand up straight (when your earlobe is directly over your instep), the natural curves of your spine are properly supported by your back muscles.

STRETCHING YOUR BACK

Stretching may ease your back pain if the problem appears to be muscular. This exercise is a simple example of the kind of stretch that is often effective. However, if you find that it aggravates the pain, do not proceed any further. If, on the other hand, the exercise does seem to help ease your back pain, perform it two to three times each day. To prepare for the exercise, apply an ice pack to the painful area for 5 minutes, or use an ice spray (available from any pharmacist) for 5–10 seconds.

1   Lie on your back, with a folded towel under your head, your knees bent, your feet flat on the floor and a hand on each knee. Breathe in, then as you exhale lightly draw your stomach down toward your spine. At the same time, pull your knees toward your shoulders (not your chest) until you feel a slight stretch (not pain) in your back. Hold, breathing normally, with your lower abdomen lightly pulled in toward your spine, for four to five breathing cycles (in and out).

2   As you exhale, draw your knees a little further toward your shoulders. Hold for up to 3 minutes, then relax with knees bent and feet flat on the floor.

Alternative: If this stretching exercise aggravates the pain, try standing as tall as you can and arching your back a little, with both hands at waist level to support you. If this makes your back feel better, do this backward stretch two to three times a day, for a minute or two at a time. It can also be easily performed lying face down on the floor or bed.

Hydrotherapy can ease back pain in several ways: ice and "warming" compresses relax tense muscles; alternate hot and cold applications improve circulation; and periodic ice applications reduce inflammation. Avoid hot packs, unless you follow up with massage or a cold application, as heat alone, even though it may feel good at the time, will usually lead to local congestion.

If your pain is being worsened by inflammation, try anti-inflammatory dietary strategies. If stress and anxiety are affecting you, relaxation methods, such as autogenic training, biofeedback and visualization may be helpful, too.

CHEST PAIN

Associated as it often is with heart conditions, chest pain can be worrying. However, pain in the chest is more likely to relate to the muscles between the ribs (the intercostal muscles), or to rib restrictions, than to the heart. If we do not breathe properly (see pages 66–74), your intercostal muscles can develop trigger points and become highly stressed, and the ribs can become limited in their range of movement. When we correct our breathing the intercostal or rib pain should ease. Angina pain (which usually manifests first in the left arm) tends to remain unaltered, even when we breathe properly. So, if you are concerned about the cause of your chest pain, inhale and exhale fully a few times – if the pain changes, your heart is probably not to blame. If you are in any doubt, consult a doctor.

> **TOP TIP** If you have a painful cough, try putting two drops of hyssop (or Olbas) oil into a bowl of hot water. With a towel covering your head and the bowl, place your face over the rising steam, and breathe slowly for 10 minutes.

Chest pain that worsens when you are resting may be caused by a digestive problem or inflammation, and you should seek medical advice. If you have chest pain without obvious cause, and you are an asthmatic, or have had a recent bout of coughing, then you can reduce your pain through a combination of massage and other bodywork; self-applied positional release methods (see pages 101–102); and stretching. Chest pain may also derive from spinal problems – these should be checked for by an appropriate practitioner.

Methods that often ease pain in tense chest muscles include TENS, acupuncture, a "warming" compress and all relaxation methods.

BLADDER, PROSTATE AND ABDOMINAL PAIN

If you feel a burning pain on urination you may have a **bladder infection**. Ultimately, you should seek advice from your doctor, who may prescribe antibiotics, but in the meantime increase your fluid intake, especially water, to not less than 4 pints (2 litres) a day and take capsules of cranberry extract or drink cranberry juice (unsugared). Cranberry contains natural chemicals that help in the elimination of bacteria from the bladder. Various herbal teas, including buchu and parsley, may also be helpful.

An **enlarged prostate** may lead to difficulty in urinating, as well as aching or burning pain on urination. Seek medical advice if you are suffering from these symptoms. Taking zinc supplements, extracts of saw palmetto berries, *Pygeum africanum* or nettle root over a period

> **TOP TIP** Hydrotherapy provides an excellent remedy for bladder, kidney and prostate problems. Try spending between 20 and 40 minutes in a "neutral" bath (see page 90), or consult an expert practitioner.

of several months may bring long-term benefit. You can derive more immediate, though temporary, relief from a prostatic massage (performed by a trained healthcare provider).

Abdominal pain can arise from so many different conditions that only general comments are possible here. These first-aid approaches should not replace responsible medical advice.

Much abdominal pain can be traced back to psychological roots. Emotional stress tends to lead to rapid, upper-chest breathing. This, in turn, means that you swallow more air, which results in bloating and sometimes the aggravation of existing abdominal pain caused by such problems as hiatus hernia. Many relaxation methods, such as progressive muscular relaxation, meditation, visualization and slow, deep (diaphragmatic) breathing can help enormously.

Many types of abdominal pain respond well to herbal remedies. For example, the antispasmodic properties of peppermint may relieve stomach cramps. This can be taken in the form of tea, drops or capsules. Try taking ginger, chamomile, aloe vera or slippery elm (as teas, extracts or powders) to treat digestive upsets. Mastic powder (derived from a resin that is produced by the shrub *Pistacia lentiscus*) is more efficient at deactivating the bacteria that cause gastric ulcers than most antibiotics. You can ease pain relating to a spastic colon by taking aloe vera juice, slippery-elm powder (mixed into a paste with water) or charcoal capsules.

A "warming" compress around the abdomen and lower chest can help to soothe stomach ache and abdominal pains in general. Or you could ask your partner or a friend to massage your back or abdomen using lavender or diluted chamomile essential oil. However, ensure that you do not massage directly over any inflamed tissues or organs.

GYNECOLOGICAL AND CHILDBIRTH PAIN

For safety, most **gynecological pain** requires medical investigation and attention, but here is a brief look at some interim, self-help measures you can try.

To ease pelvic pain and cramps, try physical and mental relaxation methods (for example, autogenic training and visualization), as well as massage, or sustained thumb or tennis-ball pressure to the lower back. Hydrotherapy methods, such as a "warming" compress on the waist, can also help, while herbal aids include black haw and cramp bark taken as tinctures (seek advice from a qualified medical herbalist) and ginger-root tea.

Chronic pelvic pain is often caused by trigger points in the lower abdominal and upper thigh muscles, as well as internally. Deactivating these points, using methods such as muscle energy technique (see pages 104–107), can often eradicate symptoms. In the USA, a group of more than 100 women with chronic pelvic pain underwent trigger-point treatment. This removed all pelvic pain from 90 percent of the women, with most pain free a year later.

If you are suffering from vaginal irritation, or pain resulting from yeast infection (thrush), try using vaginal suppositories infused with tea-tree oil or calendula; or you could mix acidophilus (a "friendly" micro-organism, available as a powder or capsule from health stores) into live yogurt and apply this mixture on a tampon. You may find that dietary strategies and supplementation (such as probiotics) help, particularly if a low-sugar diet is also followed. Consult a qualified nutritionist or naturopath for advice.

> **TOP TIP** Taking raspberry-leaf tea, an ancient folk remedy, for some days before and during delivery eases labour pain without interfering with the strength of your contractions.

Many non-pharmaceutical measures can reduce **childbirth pain**: giving birth in a water tub; acupuncture; breathing techniques (especially calming breathing, see page 72); and relaxation and visualization. Visiting an osteopath once a month in the last trimester will ease the discomfort of advanced pregnancy and help prepare your pelvis and back for childbirth. A good source of relaxation and pain relief is a "neutral" bath of no less than 20 minutes.

Your birth partner can help to ease pain during your labour by applying direct thumb pressure to tender areas of your sacrum (at the base of the spine), as well as to your back just below the lowest rib, close to the spine. You can also apply acupressure yourself. Once contractions start, try pressing firmly the tender area about one hand's width above the inner ankle bone (Spleen 6 in Chinese medicine), for up to five minutes every half hour (this point should not be stimulated before the 38th week of pregnancy). The acupressure exercise on page 152 may also help. If you are giving birth in a medical setting, such "alternative" methods will need to be discussed in advance.

BODYWIDE PAIN

Bodywide conditions demand bodywide attention – constitutional, whole-person strategies. Methods that have a calming effect on the body as a whole, such as acupuncture, relaxation massage, biofeedback, mindfulness meditation, autogenic training and breathing retraining, can alleviate – even if only temporarily – any of the conditions discussed here.

The causes of the chronic muscular-pain condition **fibromyalgia** are complex, often originating in a genetic predisposition and aggravated by one or more factors, such as trauma, a biochemical disturbance (for example, thyroid hormone imbalance) or a severe emotional upset. Central sensitization will have evolved, and strategies will be needed to avoid aggravating this further, while attempting to reduce the pain inputs from peripherally sensitized areas that feed into the sensitization process.

Treatment has to be very gentle indeed, to avoid placing new demands on already overloaded body systems. Strategies need to address the causes of fibromyalgia, as well as relieve the constant pain and fatigue that typify the condition. Apart from the general therapies mentioned above, you could try: thyroid hormone rebalancing (if appropriate, and under medical supervision); non-invasive manipulation methods, such as positional release technique (see pages 101–102); gentle and closely monitored progressive aerobic exercise; and sleep-enhancement methods.

Similar to fibromyalgia, **myofascial pain syndrome** is the result of multiple active trigger points. These can usually be deactivated by neuromuscular massage, acupuncture or dry needling methods. However, the causes of the trigger point activity also need addressing – and this usually involves paying attention to lifestyle, posture, breathing, diet and stress-related issues.

The burning, tingling or aching sensations associated with chronic **nerve pain** may derive from inflammation (neuritis), irritation or entrapment (neuralgia), or a disease of the central nervous system, such as multiple sclerosis. Other causes include infection, as in shingles, and diseases such as diabetes, cancer and arthritis. You may be able to ease nerve pain by taking supplements of vitamin B-complex, or herbs such as passiflora, valerian or Jamaican dogwood (but only in consultation with a medical herbalist).

A strategy known as counter-irritation may also help to treat nerve pain. Try rubbing an extract of cayenne pepper onto a

TOP TIP Wearing a copper bracelet can ease the pain of rheumatoid arthritis. The copper, which is absorbed through your skin, helps to protect the joint membranes and joint-lubrication fluids that are damaged by the disease.

chronically painful area – although the skin will redden, pain usually recedes noticeably. In the case of the painful scars left over after shingles, rub in an extract of red chilli peppers. Be patient, as it may take a day or two for you to feel the benefits.

Osteoarthritis is caused by wear and tear of the joints. In the early stages of the condition, you can do much to maintain good function through appropriate bodywork – stretching and movement – taking care not to irritate the joints. If you are overweight, you should lose weight, as this may be placing extra stress on your joints. You can also derive benefit from hydrotherapy (for example, compresses and Epsom-salts baths) and nutritional measures, including: reducing animal-fat intake; taking supplements of eicosapentenoic acid (EPA), glucosamine sulphate and chondroitin sulphate; and ingesting herbs such as devil's claw (in the form of dried, powdered root or as a tincture) and feverfew (eat one leaf a day).

The joint inflammation that characterizes **rheumatoid arthritis** can be eased by following a diet low in protein and sugar, but high in EPA (see pages 128–30). Other helpful treatments include TENS (at a high setting) and gentle exercise that maintains muscle tone without irritating inflamed joints.

A WORK IN PROGRESS

Planning a campaign to reduce pain demands that you understand what lies at the root of the problem. By becoming familiar with the nature, causes and usual progression of your condition, you can make informed choices about exercises, manual treatments, medication, diet, stress management and so on.

Having established a general plan in conjunction with someone objective and knowledgeable, such as a doctor or other suitably qualified healthcare provider, you need to move on to the finer points of your plan. Your pain journal will be the linchpin of any project in pain management (see box, over page). Draw up a list of action points – appointments to make with therapists or teachers, and equipment or materials to buy (for example, a TENS unit, essential oils, herbs and nutritional supplements).

So far, so good. However, you may find sticking to your plan tougher than you imagined at the initial organizational stage. After a few weeks, you may start to question what you are doing. To maintain a positive outlook, give yourself a regular pep-talk – remind yourself of your objectives, set yourself challenges, congratulate yourself on every one of your achievements – no matter how small. See over page for advice on how to monitor your progress and maintain a constant attitude of enquiry so that you can regularly re-evaluate your approach to get the best results.

Rehabilitation and recovery require time, together with focused effort to avoid aggravating matters while you try to enhance the process of healing. An understanding of the mechanisms involved helps a great deal, which is where this book, together with the further reading suggestions, can help. Only you can put all the information together in a way that is ideal for your needs, while drawing on the help that is available from others.

The road to control over your pain may seem intolerably long at times, but look how far you have come already.

LOOKING BACK AND LOOKING AHEAD

It is vital that you regularly re-evaluate your initial pain-relief plan, dropping some methods, modifying others and introducing new strategies to keep pace with changing circumstances. Review your journal at a set time each week – look out for patterns, such as particular activities that seem to raise or lower your pain scores. Change your routine accordingly. Even methods that are working well need revisiting, and possibly revitalizing, to ensure that you do not "outgrow" them. For example:

- Vary your relaxation exercises so that they do not become repetitive – introduce new ones or modify existing ones.

- Introduce fresh affirmations to reflect your evolving recovery and attitude – this will ensure that the statements continue to carry meaning for you, rather than becoming automatic.

- Once tight muscles have eased, modify your stretching exercises so that they maintain, rather than increase, muscle length.

- As your fitness improves, you should increase the intensity of your aerobic exercises – taking care not to exceed your pulse-rate limit.

- If you have excluded particular foods from your diet, reintroduce them gradually after six months to check if you have overcome your sensitivity.

- Keep up with new knowledge by reading reports, participating in online forums and discussing wider issues with friends and family.

Finally, do not underestimate the importance of your pain journal. It will become indispensable. As you look back, you will see what worked and what didn't – essential information in deciding which turn to take next in your journey toward improved health and reduced pain.

FURTHER READING

Bruce, Barbara, *Mayo Clinic Guide to Pain Relief*, Mayo Clinic Health
Solutions: Rochester, 2008

Chaitow, Leon, *Fibromyalgia and Muscle Pain*, Thorsons: London,
2011 (new edition)

— *Maintaining Body Balance, Flexibility & Stability*, Churchill
Livingstone: Philadelphia, 2003

Davies, Clair, Davies, Amber and Simons, David, G., *The Trigger
Point Therapy Workbook*, New Harbinger Publications: Oakland,
2004 (second edition)

DeLaune, Valerie, *Trigger Point Therapy for Headaches and
Migraines*, New Harbinger Publications: Oakland, 2008

Gloth III, F. Michael, *Handbook of Pain Relief in Older Adults* (Aging
Medicine), Humana Press: New York, 2010 (second edition)

Kabat-Zinn, Jon, *Mindfulness Meditation for Pain Relief*, Sounds True:
2009 (Audio CD)

Lewandowski, Michael J., *The Chronic Pain Care Workbook*, New
Harbinger Publications: Oakland, 2006

Schatz, Mary Pullig, Iyengar, B.K.S. and Connor, William, *Back Care
Basics: A Doctor's Gentle Yoga Program for Back and Neck Pain
Relief*, Rodmell Press: Berkeley, 1992

Shlomo, Vaknin, Yourell, Robert A. and Raz, Arin, *Pain Away:
Advanced Mental Techniques for Immediate & Long Lasting Relief*,
Inner Patch Publishing: Prague, 2010

Stone, Victoria, *The World's Best Massage Techniques*, Fair Winds
Press: Minneapolis, 2010

Wise, David and Anderson, Rodney, *Headache in the Pelvis*, National
Center for Pelvic Pain Research: Occidental, 2010 (sixth revised
edition)

REFERENCES

UNDERSTANDING YOUR PAIN

[1] Butler, D. and Moseley L., *Explain Pain*, NOI Group Publishing: Adelaide, 2003

[2] Kindler, L. et al, "Risk factors predicting the development of widespread pain from chronic back or neck pain", *Journal of Pain* 11(12) (2010): 1320–28

[3] Woolf, C., "Central sensitization: Implications for the diagnosis and treatment of pain", *Biennial Review of Pain* 152(3) (2011): S2–15

[4] Nijls, J. et al, "Recognition of central sensitization in patients with musculoskeletal pain: Application of pain neurophysiology in manual therapy practice", *Man Ther* 15 (2010): 135–41

[5] Affaitati, G., Costantini, R., Fabrizio A. et al, "Effects of treatment of peripheral pain generators in fibromyalgia patients", *European Journal of Pain* 15(1) (2011): 61–9

[6] Ge, H.Y. et al, "Contribution of the local and referred pain from active myofascial trigger points in fibromyalgia syndrome", *Pain* 147 (2009): 233–40

[7] Rennefeld, C. et al, "Habituation to pain: Further support for a central component", *Pain* 148(3) (2010): 503–8

POSITIVE ATTITUDES

[1] Baudic, S. et al "Interaction between apathy and mental flexibility on pain coping strategies in fibromyalgia", Poster Sessions / *European Journal of Pain* 13 (2009): S55–285

[2] Farber, E. et al, "Resilience factors associated with adaptation to HIV disease", *Psychosomatics* 41 (2000): 140–46

[3] Finer, B., "People in pain", *Pain* 121(1–2) (2006): 168

[4] West, C. et al, "Family resilience: Towards a new model of chronic pain management", *Collegian* 18 (2011): 3–10

[5] **Walsh, F.,** *Strengthening Family Resilience*, The Guilford Press: New York, 2006 (second edition)

[6] **Vance, C.,** "Enhance patient compliance by targeting different learning styles", *Podiatry Today*, 16(8) (2003): 28–9

FINDING PEACE

[1] **Glazer, H.I.,** "Dysesthetic vulvodynia: Long-term follow-up after treatment with surface electromyography-assisted pelvic floor muscle rehabilitation", *J. Reprod. Med* 45 (2000): 798–802

COMPLEMENTARY THERAPIES

[1] **Cao, H. et al,** "Medicinal cupping therapy in 30 patients with fibromyalgia: A case series observation", *Forsch Komplementmed* 18(3) (2011): 122–6

[2] **Montes-Molina, R. et al,** "Interferential laser therapy in the treatment of shoulder pain and disability from musculoskeletal pathologies: A randomised comparative study", *Physiotherapy* (2011). Article in press.

[3] **Somboonwong, J., et al,** "The therapeutic efficacy and properties of topical Aloe vera in thermal burns", *Journal of the Medical Association of Thailand* 87(4) (2004): 69–78

[4] **Adkison, J.,** "The effect of topical arnica on muscle pain", *The Annals of Pharmacotherapy* 44(10) (2010): 1579–84

[5] **Cichoke, A.,** "The use of proteolytic enzymes with soft tissue athletic injuries", American Chiropractor (1981): 32

[6] **Gagnier, J. et al,** "Herbal medicine for low back pain: A Cochrane review", *Spine* 32(1) (2007): 82–92

[7] **Srivastava, J. et al,** "Health promoting benefits of chamomile in the elderly population" in *Complementary and Alternative Therapies and the Aging Population*, Elsevier: Oxford, 2009

[8] **Chaieb, K. et al,** "The chemical composition and biological activity of clove essential oil, Eugenia caryophyllata (Syzigium aromaticum L. Myrtaceae): A short review", *Phytotherapy Research* 21(6) (2007): 501–506

[9] **Giannetti, B. et al,** "Efficacy and safety of comfrey root extract ointment in the treatment of acute upper or lower back pain: Results of a double-blind, randomised, placebo controlled, multicentre trial", *British Journal of Sports Medicine* 44(9) (2010): 637–41

[10] **Romm, A., et al** "Menstrual wellness and menstrual problems" in *Botanical Medicine for Women's Health*, Elsevier: Edinburgh, 2010, 97–185

[11] **Reyes-Gordillo, K.,** "Curcumin protects against acute liver damage in the rat by inhibiting NF-kappaB, proinflammatory cytokines production and oxidative stress", *Biochimica et Biophysica Acta,* 1770(6) (2007): 989–96

[12] **Warnock, M.,** "Effectiveness and safety of Devil's Claw tablets in patients with general rheumatic disorders", *Phytotherapy Research* 21(12) (2007): 1228–33

[13] **Grzanna, R.,** "Ginger: An herbal medicinal product with broad anti-inflammatory actions", *Journal of Medicinal Food* 8(2) (2005): 125–32

[14] **Dillard, J., Knapp, S.,** "Complementary and alternative pain therapy in the emergency department, *Emergency Medicine Clinics of North America* 23(2) (2005): 529

[15] **Vakilian K. et al,** Healing advantages of lavender essential oil during episiotomy recovery: A clinical trial", *Complementary Therapies in Clinical Practice* 17(1) (2011): 50–53

[16] **Galeotti, N., et al,** "St. John's Wort reduces neuropathic pain through a hypericin-mediated inhibition of the protein kinase C γ and ε activity", *Biochemical Pharmacology* 79(9) (2010): 1327–36

[17] **Bashir, S. et al**, "Studies on the antioxidant and analgesic activities of Aztec marigold (Tagetes erecta) flowers", *Phytotherapy Research* 22(12) (2008): 1692–4

[18] **Beer, A.,** "Willow bark extract (Salicis cortex) for gonarthrosis and coxarthrosis: Results of a cohort study with a control group", *Phytomedicine,* 15(11) (2008): 907

EATING WELL

[1] **Li S., Micheletti, R.,** "Role of diet in rheumatic disease", *Rheumatic Disease Clinics of North America* 37(1) (2011): 119–33

[2] **Beauchamp, G. et al,** "Phytochemsitry: Ibuprofen-like activity in extra-virgin olive oil", *Nature* 437 (2005): 45–6

[3] **Juge-Aubry, C. et al,** "Adipose tissue: A regulator of inflammation", *Best Practice & Research Clinical Endocrinology & Metabolism* 19(4) (2005): 547–66

[4] **Berg, A., Scherer P.,** "Adipose tissue, inflammation, and cardiovascular disease", *Circulation Research* 96 (2005): 939

[5] **Esposito, K. et al,** "Effect of a Mediterranean-style diet on endothelial dysfunction and markers of vascular inflammation in the metabolic syndrome", *Journal of the American Medical Association* 292(12) (2004): 1440–46

[6] **Alpay, K. et al,** "Diet restriction in migraine, based on IgG against foods: A clinical double-blind, randomised, cross-over trial", *Cephalalgia* 30(7) (2010): 829–37

TYPES OF PAIN

[1] **Rozen, T. et al,** "Open label trial of coenzyme Q10 as a migraine preventive", *Cephalalgia* 22(2) (2002):137–41

INDEX

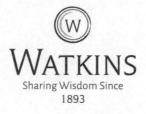

WATKINS
Sharing Wisdom Since
1893

The story of Watkins dates back to 1893, when the scholar of esotericism John Watkins founded a bookshop, inspired by the lament of his friend and teacher Madame Blavatsky that there was nowhere in London to buy books on mysticism, occultism or metaphysics. That moment marked the birth of Watkins, soon to become the home of many of the leading lights of spiritual literature, including Carl Jung, Rudolf Steiner, Alice Bailey and Chögyam Trungpa.

Today, the passion at Watkins Publishing for vigorous questioning is still resolute. Our wide-ranging and stimulating list reflects the development of spiritual thinking and new science over the past 120 years. We remain at the cutting edge, committed to publishing books that change lives.

DISCOVER MORE . . .

Read our blog

Watch and listen to
our authors in action

Sign up to
our mailing list

JOIN IN THE CONVERSATION

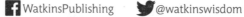

f WatkinsPublishing **🐦** @watkinswisdom

▶ watkinsbooks **📷** watkinswisdom **☁** watkins-media

Our books celebrate conscious, passionate, wise and happy living.
Be part of the community by visiting

www.watkinspublishing.com